George E. Berkley, Ph.D., is a social scientist who has long been following developments in the field of preventive health care. He is affiliated with Boston State College.

Robert D. Vachon, M.D., who wrote the foreword, is medical director of Nasson College in Springvale, Maine. He is a member of the International Academy of Preventive Medicine.

CANCER

HOW TO PREVENT IT
&
HOW TO HELP YOUR DOCTOR FIGHT IT

George E. Berkley, Ph.D.
Foreword: Robert D. Vachon, M.D.

A SPECTRUM BOOK

Prentice-Hall, Inc., *Englewood Cliffs, New Jersey 07632*

Library of Congress Cataloging in Publication Data

BERKLEY, GEORGE E.
    Cancer.

    (A Spectrum Book)
    Bibliography: p.
    Includes index.
    1. Cancer—Prevention.   2. Cancer—
Nutritional aspects.   3. Orthomolecular
medicine.   I. Title.
RC268.B47   616.9'94   77-26954
ISBN 0-13-113399-3
ISBN 0-13-113381-0 pbk.

A SPECTRUM BOOK

Printed in the United States of America

10   9   8   7   6   5   4   3   2

PRENTICE-HALL INTERNATIONAL, INC., *London*
PRENTICE-HALL OF AUSTRALIA PTY. LIMITED, *Sydney*
PRENTICE-HALL OF CANADA, LTD., *Toronto*
PRENTICE-HALL OF INDIA PRIVATE LIMITED, *New Delhi*
PRENTICE-HALL OF JAPAN, INC., *Tokyo*
PRENTICE-HALL OF SOUTHEAST ASIA PTE. LTD., *Singapore*
WHITEBALL BOOKS LIMITED, *Wellington, New Zealand*

What though the radiance which was once so bright
Be now for ever taken from my sight,
     though nothing can bring back the hour
Of splendour in the grass, of glory in the flower
     We will grieve not, rather find
     strength in what remains behind.

WORDSWORTH

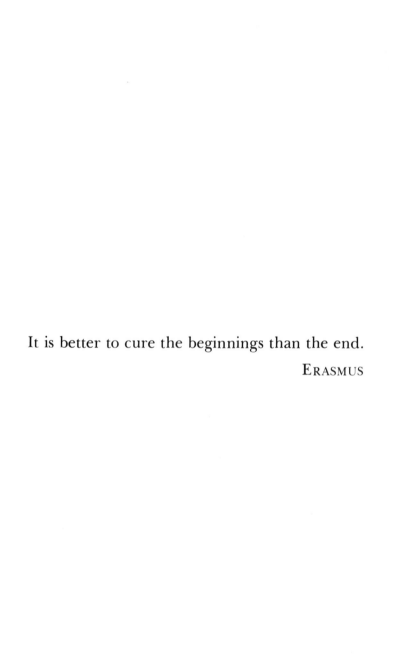

It is better to cure the beginnings than the end.

ERASMUS

Contents

Foreword

Modern medicine is often an either-or proposition. The patient either has pneumonia or he doesn't. He either needs an appendectomy or he doesn't. Situations such as these provide the practicing physician with little time or opportunity to make the type of assessments or evaluations upon which preventive medicine must be based. Nutritional deficiencies, for example, may lead to many kinds of illnesses, but too often the physician does not know about such deficiencies until the illness occurs. And sometimes not even then.

Let me offer an example. A medical team at Johns Hopkins University Hospital examined the cases of sixty-nine deceased patients whose autopsies had disclosed that they had suffered from scurvy. The team found that the attending physician had diagnosed the disease in only six of these cases.

To some extent this reflects the lack of instruction given

to physicians in nutrition. Only 24 percent of American medical schools currently offer any courses in this subject. And, to some extent, the failure to make the appropriate diagnosis may stem from the fact that outright scurvy, which results from a deficiency of vitamin C, has become relatively rare in the United States. But this incident also reveals the neglected nature of dietary diagnosis. Too often the malnourished patient may be feeling neither completely well nor completely ill, and such a condition could last for years.

Fortunately, the situation seems to be slowly changing—physicians, as well as other health professionals, appear to be increasingly aware that there is much more to medicine than simply diagnosing an apparent illness and prescribing a cure.

As an example of what I mean, let us take a look at an experiment that was carried out at the tumor clinic of the University of Alabama Medical Center in 1966. Some fifty-four women suffering from cervical cancer were scheduled for radiation treatment at the clinic. One week before the start of the treatment, half of these patients were put on a special hypernutritional diet. The other twenty-seven were given no special nutritional treatment or advice. Three weeks after the termination of radiation therapy, the women who had not received any special nutritional help showed a response rate of 63.3 percent, which is normal for such treatment. However, the experimental group who received the special diet displayed a response rate of 97.5 percent.

If one week of good nutrition can affect cancer recovery to such an extent, think of the role that good nutrition can play in the overall cancer problem!

In recent years much material has come to light regarding the importance that nutritional, psychological, and other factors can have in the formation, or, as the case may be, the prevention, of cancer. Doctor Berkley has ably put much of this material into a form in which it can be easily understood

and easily utilized by the layman. As a physician whose practice for thirty-five years has been oriented to preventive
medicine, I recommend this book to all those concerned
about cancer. And with the cancer rate continuing to climb,
that should include just about everyone.

ROBERT D. VACHON, M.D.

Preface

In writing prefaces most writers thank their wives for their solace and support only after thanking everyone else. I should like to reverse that order here for my wife, Patricia, aided and abetted this project from the very beginning. She fully shared my conviction that the public desperately needs the largely ignored research that this book seeks to publicize. For such support, as for as many other things, I owe her an ever-mounting debt of gratitude.

I am also grateful to Dr. Robert D. Vachon, who wrote the foreword, and to the three other physicians who read, in whole or in part, the initial draft of the manuscript; their suggestions were most helpful.

The need to incorporate their suggestions plus the need to keep abreast of such a rapidly developing field forced me to make revisions in the text up to the last minute. However, since lack of time made it impossible to blend all the new material into the text itself, I have placed much of it in the bibliographical notes and comments at the end. Consequently, although this section was initially designed merely to provide annotation for students and practitioners in the health care system, it now contains much other material as well. As a result, more interested lay readers may also wish to glance at it.

I also wish to thank Prentice-Hall field editor Paul Misselwitch for spotting the manuscript and Prentice-Hall Spectrum editor Lynne Lumsden for shepherding it through to publication.

And I would also like to express my appreciation for, and my amazement at, the way Mrs. Marie Shinkwin transformed my smeared and scratchy scrawl into neatly typed and letter-perfect copy.

Finally, although the book is dedicated to my aunt who died suddenly of cancer in the fall of 1976, it was the previous contracting of cancer by my mother-in-law, Mrs. Margaret Aggett, that first inspired me to write it. The effect of her subsequent death on her husband, Albert, on my wife, and on all the many others who knew and loved her spurred on this effort to help spare other families from similar and, so I believe, largely unnecessary tragedies.

1

A Peril and a Hope

In 1968 a group of surgeons examined a patient on whom they had recently performed a kidney transplant. The operation had gone quite smoothly, and they anticipated no ill effects from what had become, by this time, an almost routine, albeit delicate, piece of surgery. They were thus completely unprepared for what they saw.

The upper half of the kidney had grown to three times the size of the lower half. Furthermore, an X ray of the patient showed that he had developed a mass on his chest. Without knowing it they had transplanted a cancerous kidney. And the cancer was now starting to spread to the rest of the recipient's body.

By removing the diseased kidney and placing the patient on chronic dialysis instead, they were able to arrest the cancer and save the man's life. But the question remained: why had the *donor* of the kidney never shown signs of having cancer? Why had the cancer remained arrested when the kidney was in the donor's body only to become activated when it was transplanted into another human being?

Some other discoveries about this time were also causing conjecture. Surgeons doing postmortems were finding signs of cancer in some of their cadavers. Yet these were the bodies of people who had given no indication of harboring such malignancies when alive and had died of other causes. For some reason or other, their cancers had remained confined to the point where neither they nor their doctors had ever noticed them.

A new theory had arisen to explain such mysterious occurrences. Developed by the Australian physician Burnet, it was based on the workings of the body's immunization system. Medicine had long known that human beings, like other animals, manage to mobilize defenses against external attack. Thus, when a person receives a cut on the hand, say, the white corpuscles tend to multiply in order to ward off infection. The human being's defense system does not always win, of course, but it always succeeds in staging some sort of a fight.

Burnett postulated that our immunization system protects us not only from outside aggressors, but from internal ones as well. The human body, so it seems, reproduces billions of cells a day. In so doing, it cannot avoid making many errors. Fortunately, in most of us most of the time, the immunization system quickly stamps out these abnormal cells. However, when the system becomes weak or otherwise deficient, the abnormal cells grow and spread, becoming the cancers that now strike one out of every four Americans.

The immunization theory explains why arrested states of cancer can turn up in the corpses of people who, during their lifetimes, seemed never to suffer from the disease. It also explains why the transplanted cancerous kidney started to take off, as it were, once it found a new home. In preparing a patient for a kidney transplant, physicians always suppress his immunization system so that his body will not reject the new organ. In so doing in this case, they gave the disease free rein to roam throughout the man's body.

The immunization theory opens up a whole new way of viewing cancer. It strongly suggests that all of us come into constant contact with at least the very preliminary stages of the disease. The one thousand Americans who die every day from the malignancy do not really "catch" cancer. Rather, they are simply the ones who are unable to annihilate or at least arrest it.

The theory also explains why conventional efforts at controlling cancer have borne so little fruit. The death rates from those contracting the most common forms of cancer have remained about the same for the past twenty-five years. Organized medicine so far has largely devoted its attention to finding a cure for cancer rather than directing its enormous research expenditures—currently at the rate of nearly one billion dollars a year—to finding ways to improve the human body's own immunization system.

Fortunately, some medical practitioners, including some of the very best, have viewed the disease from this perspective all along. In choosing to march to a different drummer, they have built up a remarkably impressive, though regrettably little known, body of evidence. Their evidence supports and strengthens the immunization theory. More importantly, this evidence, taken in toto, clearly indicates that

1. Most people can avoid cancer by taking a few rather simple, largely dietary precautions.
2. Most people who do suffer from the disease can greatly increase their chances of survival through the same means.

The above statements may strike you, to say nothing of your doctor, as rash and ridiculous, if not downright false and fraudulent. But before passing judgment, I invite you, as well as your doctor, to look at the research that supports them. And let us start by looking at the record of the first doctor who used the immunization theory approach and the device of diet to fight cancer. This physician's name was Dr. Max Gerson.

2

The Case of
Dr. Gerson

If in the 1920s you asked a German doctor who was his country's greatest surgeon, he almost certainly would have responded with the name of Ferdinand Sauerbruch. After all, it was Sauerbruch who had performed the first successful operation on the human heart, Sauerbruch who had pioneered in thoracic surgery, Sauerbruch who received invitations to speak at medical conferences everywhere.

It was while traveling by train en route to one of these conferences that Sauerbruch made a startling discovery. He was sharing a compartment with a fidgety passenger whose face bore the telltale signs of scar tissue. Sauerbruch guessed that the man had once suffered some bad burns. Not at all, replied his fellow traveler, the scars were from skin tuberculosis.

Sauerbruch refused to believe the man's story. Skin tuberculosis, known medically as lupus vulgaris, was at that time incurable, even untreatable. "There is no cure for lupus," the great surgeon snorted. But the man insisted that he had had it. Sauerbruch proceeded then and there to unfasten the man's jacket and shirt and to give him an impromptu examination. To his great surprise, he saw on his fellow passenger's chest large areas of perfectly healed skin tuberculosis.

The man attributed this medical miracle to a young internist in Bielefeld named Max Gerson. And the means Dr. Gerson used, he said, was diet. Sauerbruch asked him to bring the internist to see him in Munich. The passenger obliged, and two weeks later Sauerbruch, as he related it in his book *Master Surgeon*, found sitting across his desk "a modest man with an intelligent face." It was Dr. Gerson.

Gerson told the master surgeon that he himself had once suffered from severe migraine headaches. In his depression to find a cure he had tried changing his diet and eventually had come across a regimen that cured him. He then proceeded to use the same technique on patients suffering the same problem. The results were almost uniformly successful. Then, by chance, one patient found that the Gerson diet also cured his skin tuberculosis as well. Since that time, the internist had been prescribing his cure for sufferers of this disease, and the results were almost uniformly excellent.

What was this special diet that yielded such remarkable results? It was simply a diet that excluded all salt.

Sauerbruch reacted initially with some degree of skepticism and scorn. He could see no relationship between such a treatment and such a cure. But since he had seen one instance of proof in his fellow train passenger, he decided to put the treatment to a test.

He set up a wing of his clinic as a "lupus station" and found 450 patients willing to try out the treatment. The initial results were disappointing. Though not a grain of salt went into the patients' food, the disease continued to ravage their skin. Then, Sauerbruch found out by accident that an overly sympathetic nurse had taken to smuggling in sausages, beer, and other taboo items to the deprived patients.

Sauerbruch resumed the test under more carefully controlled conditions. And, as he related it, "Soon, Dr. Gerson was proved right. Nearly all our patients recovered; their sores almost disappeared under our very eyes. In this experiment involving 450 patients, only four could not be cured by Dr. Gerson's saltless diet." The Gerson diet had been proven to be over 99% effective.

Gerson's fame began to spread. Articles about him started to appear in the popular press and patients flocked to his door. The Weimar Republic, on his advice, began using dehydrated food instead of canned goods to feed its army. The German medical establishment, however, was not pleased. Except for Sauerbruch and a few others, most of the country's leading practitioners denounced the Gerson method as not scientific.

A demonstration was finally arranged to take place at the Berlin Medical School in May of 1933. However, Hitler came to power in the interim and Dr. Gerson, who was Jewish, found himself forced to flee to Austria in March. After practicing in Vienna, where he again encountered the hostility of the medical fraternity, now aided and abetted by a rising tide of anti-Semitism, he left for Paris. In the French capital, one of his former patients, who was president of the Banque de Paris, set him up in a clinic. But soon he left Paris to come to New York, where he became licensed to practice medicine in 1938.

Over the years Gerson began using his dietary methods to treat other human ailments. In 1928 he used it to cure a case of cancer of the bile ducts. He then applied it to twelve more cancer cases and obtained, so he later claimed, seven successes. In Vienna he administered a modification of the diet to six cancer patients with no results. In Paris he treated seven more cancer cases. Three, he said, turned out favorably, while one remained undecided. In 1941 he began treating cancer on a regular basis in New York and in a live-in clinic he established on Long Island.

Gerson's anticancer diet, like his antilupus diet, was salt-free. It was also designed to be fat-free. It concentrated on building up potassium in the system instead. The patient lived largely on fruit and vegetable juices and on a soup made from parsley roots, celery knobs, leeks, tomatoes, onions, potatoes, and carrots. The cancer sufferer was also given Lugol's solution for iodine, brewer's yeast, liver shots, and some other supplements. He was even taught to give the liver injections to himself. Some oatmeal was also permitted.

The diet forbade alcohol, tobacco, white flour, meat, and fish, especially when smoked, canned, or preserved in any way. Chocolate, coffee, tea, and spices were also taboo. Proteins were largely excluded, and most medications were also disallowed. Gerson particularly warned against the use of anesthesia, saying that the body through his diet became so hypersensitive that an anesthesia could prove fatal.

Unpalatable as the diet may seem, it was perhaps not the most unpleasant part of the Gerson treatment. Gerson believed in the efficacy of generous bowel movements, and so frequent enemas became part of the patient's daily life.

Such a dietary and colonic schedule was obviously not designed or destined to attract patients until they had exhausted all other forms of treatment. And, as it happens, most of the afflicted who crossed his threshold were already at death's door. Their own doctors had pronounced them incurable, and they had turned to Gerson as a desperate last resort.

How well did they fare at Gerson's hands? Most of them failed to find the miracle they were seeking. But a sizable number recovered. For some, at least, the Gerson treatment worked.

Gerson himself was always the first to admit that his method was ineffective in many cases. These included those with a low blood count as well as those who suffered severe liver damage. Nevertheless, he claimed to cure 30 percent of his "hopeless" cases and nearly all those who came to him at an earlier stage.

In support of his claim, five of these "hopeless" cases appeared at a Senate subcommittee hearing in Washington in 1946, at which Gerson himself testified. The subcommittee, chaired by Senator Claude Pepper of Florida, was weighing a proposal to appropriate $100 million for cancer research. Gerson was appearing in order to support the bill, though he was not seeking any of the research funds for himself.

Gerson later presented five other successfully treated cases at a luncheon of two hundred business executives in New York City. And in a book entitled *A Cancer Therapy— Results of Fifty Cases,* he detailed his successful treatment of different types of severe malignancy.

S. J. Haught, a New York newspaper reporter, started investigating Gerson thinking the doctor was a quack. He changed his mind after he interviewed some of these patients. One was a Maywood, New Jersey, barber who had developed a tumor on his left lung. It had reached the stage where he could not even turn his neck without great pain, and his doctor had given him only a few days to live. Under the Gerson diet he had made an almost complete recovery— some muscle damage remained—and was operating a family business in Maywood when Haught interviewed him some years later.

Another case involved a soldier with a brain tumor. The tumor had been operated upon but had come back. The soldier refused a second operation and turned to Gerson. In a few months the tumor completely disappeared.

The soldier subsequently sent his sister-in-law to Gerson.

She was suffering from an ovarian tumor that would not prove fatal if operated upon, but would prevent her from having children. Gerson cured her without surgery. Several years later she returned to her original doctor with two children in tow. When the physician complimented her on adopting the youngsters, she proudly replied that they were her own. The doctor refused to believe her, but when she challenged him to call the maternity wing of Christ's Hospital in Jersey City, he did so and found that she was speaking the truth.

Gerson's most famous patient was John Gunther, Jr., the son of the author of the celebrated *Inside* books which crowded the best-seller lists during the 1930s, '40s, and '50s. The seventeen-year-old youngster began suffering from a brain tumor in 1945. His anguished father sought the help of every celebrated cancer specialist in the country. They tried all the conventional forms of treatment including surgery and X rays as well as an unconventional method involving the use of mustard. But the tumor only grew bigger.

Gunther heard about Gerson and asked the boy's doctors whether he should try him. The chief physician offered no objection, being quite certain, as he put it, that the youth would probably not last the week. One specialist recalled that the boy's polymorphonuclear blood count was down to 3 percent, indicating a profound anemia. He had never known of a recovery from such a blood condition.

This was the boy's condition and his doctors' prognosis when he was taken to Gerson in September 1946. What happened? Here is how Gunther himself put it in his moving memoir *Death Be Not Proud*. "Within a week, Johnny was feeling not worse, but much better! The blood count rose steadily, the bruises were absorbed with extraordinary speed, the wound in the bulge healed, and, miracle of miracles, the bump on the skull was going down." By the end of the month the bump had shrunk still more while the boy's blood count had risen to normal. Said Gunther, "I was beside myself with a violent and incredulous joy."

Now began a series of events whose implications and even sequence becomes difficult to pinpoint with precision from Gunther's account. Apparently the youngster continued to improve but the bump started to grow again. There were continued battles between Gerson and the other doctors over whether or not to drain it. Gerson feared any anesthesia but relented enough to allow a novocaine injection. Later he permitted hormone treatments. Meanwhile the patient had started to go steadily downhill. Another operation failed.

By this time he was out of Gerson's hands and off the Gerson diet. Gunther and his ex-wife decided to try once again the things they had tried before, starting with X ray treatments, then the mustard therapy, saving the Gerson diet for last since it was so unpleasant. However, Johnny never got a chance to go back on the diet. He died on July 1, 1947.

Gerson subsequently blamed the hormone treatments for Johnny's relapse and expressed to Haught his resentment at himself for having consented to them. However, according to Gunther's account, the downturn in the youth's condition seemed to have occurred before that time. Be that as it may, there is no question that the youth's immediate response to the Gerson treatment was strikingly positive, and a boy who was not expected to survive the week lived eight months. Moreover, noted Gunther, "I did learn beyond reasonable doubt that his [Gerson's] diet did effect other cures . . . some of his results have been astonishing."

Gerson's fights with the cancer specialists over Johnny's treatment were nothing new. The same resistance that he had encountered from his fellow physicians in Europe had arisen to confront him in America. And here there was no Sauerbruch to shield him.

The Medical Society of the County of New York

frowned on Gerson's methods and accused him of purporting to have a cancer cure, but refusing to publish his work or to demonstrate it for his colleagues. However, Haught found that Gerson had submitted articles to the recognized journals and had offered to demonstrate. All his articles and demonstration offers were rejected. (As it happens, however, Gerson had published about fifty medical papers, many of them in German journals.)

Doctors from the medical society, Haught said in his interesting and informative book *Has Dr. Max Gerson a True Cancer Cure?*, visited Gerson five times. Each time the internist showed them records, X rays, and even patients. They thanked him and left, but never issued a report on what they found. However, the pressure continued. In 1950 Gothem Hospital severed his affiliation. Finally, in 1958 the county medical society suspended his membership. The cause? He had appeared as a guest on an all-night radio talk show and thereby was guilty of "personal publicity."

Probing a little deeper, Haught found that other M.D.'s had also appeared on the talk show, which was hosted by "Long John" Nebel, but they had received no reprimands for doing so. Furthermore, Gerson's appearance had been arranged by a group of ex-patients. Finally, Dr. Gerson had no need of personal publicity, since he already had more patients than he could handle.

The medical society's pressure, however, took its toll. He was unable to secure young doctors to assist him. One result was that the overworked physician contracted pneumonia at the age of seventy-seven and died. The second result was that he left no other physicians behind who were thoroughly trained to carry on his work. The Gerson diet died with its originator, although similar cures are still being carried on by certain physicians in Europe.

Why was the medical fraternity so hostile to Gerson and his work? A statement from one of the doctors who treated

Johnny Gunther and whom the elder Gunther quotes in his books suggests a partial answer. Said this cancer specialist, "If this thing [the Gerson diet] works, we can chuck millions of dollars worth of equipment in the river and get rid of cancer by cooking carrots in a pot." Gerson and his diet were threatening the whole basis of modern medical practice.

Nevertheless, Gerson was not without collegial supporters. Five physicians submitted statements at the hearings of the Senate subcommittee testifying that they had seen Gerson achieve startling results through the use of his technique. Unfortunately, his most famous collegial backer was far away in the jungles of Africa. This was the missionary-doctor and humanist Albert Schweitzer. Dr. Schweitzer had turned to Gerson when neither he nor any of the doctors he consulted could cure Mrs. Schweitzer of tuberculosis, which was threatening to stamp out her life. After being treated by Gerson, she lived another thirty years, dying at the age of seventy-nine.

Schweitzer subsequently served as a director of the Foundation for Cancer Treatment, an organization set up by ex-patients and admirers of Gerson to further his work. And on the occasion of Gerson's death, Schweitzer wrote a lengthy letter to his fellow physician's daughter, saying, "I see in him one of the most eminent medical geniuses in the history of medicine. He possessed something elemental. Out of the deepest thought about the nature of disease and the process of healing, he came to walk along new paths with great success."

Was Gerson a medical genius? Much of the research that has come to light since his time indicates that he may not have fully understood all he was doing. For example, the lack of salt in his diet may, as we shall later see, have played less of a role in the effectiveness of his treatment than the liver shots that he administered simply to provide some basic nourishment. His emphasis on enemas may not have been all that necessary. Indeed, the findings that we now possess concerning nutrition and cancer suggest that he could have devised a diet that might have been much more palatable and more effective at the same time.

But there is no disputing the fact that Gerson was on the right track. The details of his diet aside, even the effectiveness of his treatment aside, Gerson did blaze a new trail. His approach distinctly anticipated the immunization theory that conventional medicine would discover, with much hoopla, many decades after Gerson was preaching and practicing it.

In the chapters to follow we will come across material that will incline us to modify and alter many of the specifics of the Gerson method. But all of this material will bolster and buttress his basic contention: normal healthy metabolism knows no cancer.

3

Toward the

Glasgow Experiment

Dr. Frederick Klenner was sitting in his Reidsville, North Carolina, office one day when a man burst in and gasped out the news that he was dying. It seems that the fellow had just been bitten by a huge insect ten minutes before. He was suffering severe chest pains and couldn't breathe.

Thinking that a black widow spider had inflicted the injury, Klenner quickly gave him an injection of calcium gluconate. The shot produced no effect, and the man started to turn blue from lack of oxygen. He was, quite literally, dying before the doctor's eyes.

Klenner then filled his syringe with 50,000 milligrams of vitamin C and plunged it into the victim's arm. Before he had finished the injection, the man had begun to breathe easier. In a few minutes he was able to leave, purged of the poison that had almost taken his life. "Except for vitamin C," Klenner later recalled, "the individual would have died from shock and asphyxiation."

A fluke? A mere oddity of nature? Or perhaps a mere question of mind over matter, the patient responding to the treatment simply because it was treatment? Or maybe the good doctor is just pulling our leg or imagining things?

Yet if any of these explanations are true, how then does one explain an experience that occurred some twenty years later to Dr. Gloria Williamson, assistant professor of health at North Texas State University? Dr. Williamson went out of her house one day to find that her dog had been bitten by a poisonous snake. The swelling had already spread from the paw to the shoulder and was threatening to terminate the pet's life. She hastily gave the dog 12,000 milligrams of vitamin C—an enormous amount for a dog, especially since dogs, like most animals (man is a notable exception), can and do make their own vitamin C. She followed this up with 6,000 milligrams of vitamin C every hour for six hours. The swelling began to subside, starting from the time she administered the first batch of the vitamin. Twenty-four hours after the incident took place, the animal "was as good as new."

Actually, vitamin C had hardly been discovered at the start of the 1930s when reports of its efficacy in counteracting medical malignancies had begun to appear. In 1935, for instance, Claus W. Jungeblut of Columbia University reported finding that monkeys inoculated with poliomyelitis virus failed to become paralyzed if they had been given large quantities of vitamin C. His remarkable research would seem to have opened up a whole new method for preventing this dread disease, which had afflicted numerous sufferers, including the then-president of the United States. Yet, the medical profession, in what we will continually see to be its characteristic stance, chose to ignore Jungeblut's findings and their possible implications for polio prevention.

Jungeblut continued experimenting with the vitamin, and in 1937 he reported finding that vitamin C, when put into a test tube containing tetanus toxin, would inactivate the toxin. A 1939 experiment showed that the mysterious vitamin would have the same effect on whooping cough bacteria. Further research in the 1940s showed that it would control other nasty germs such as *Proteus vulgaris* and group A hemolytic *Streptococci*.

All of this research, however, had been conducted in the laboratory. What was needed, of course, was working physicians ready to test the vitamin's effectiveness with actual patients. Finally, in the late forties, the studious silence with which the medical profession had greeted these findings was broken. Working out of his Reidsville office, Dr. Klenner became the first practicing American physician to put vitamin C to use as a therapeutic device.

Klenner had become interested in vitamin C after he had found that he could detect no signs of the vitamin in the blood or urine of people suffering from infections. Even after giving them what he then considered to be substantial amounts of the vitamin, he could still find no traces of it in their bodies. He drew from this experiment an important conclusion: vitamin C was being used to fight the infection. This conclusion led easily to another: greatly increased amounts of vitamin C would help the patient in waging this fight.

Dr. Klenner then began to use massive doses of vitamin C to treat encephalitis, meningitis, polio, viral pneumonia, tetanus, and other infections. He would usually give continuous intravenous injections of large amounts—two to four thousand milligrams—with one gram of calcium gluconate. Soon he was reporting rewarding results.

A woman suffering from pneumonia was given 140,000 milligrams of vitamin C. She recovered completely in seventy-two hours. People suffering from burns were also given high amounts while their charred skin was sprayed with a 3 percent ascorbic acid (vitamin C) solution. The burns healed much better. Diabetics given vitamin C, said Klenner, were able to utilize insulin better. Given to pregnant women, vitamin C helped maintain hemoglobin levels, greatly reduced leg cramps, and improved the capacity of the skin to resist the pressure of an expanding uterus, thereby leading to shorter and smoother labor. Of the three hundred obstetrical cases he saw treated with vitamin C, none suffered postpartem hemorrhage and none required catheterization. Failure to use adequate amounts of vitamin C in pregnancy, concluded Dr. Klenner, "verges on malpractice." (On October 13, 1973, the British medical magazine *Lancet* published a report by English researchers claiming that all pregnant women should take at least 500 milligrams a day.)

One of Klenner's most startling cases concerned an eighteen-month-old baby girl suffering from polio. The infant had become paralyzed following a convulsion, and her body had turned blue, stiff, and cold when her desperate mother brought her to his office. As a matter of fact, the physician could distinguish neither a heart nor a pulse beat; he realized she was still alive only when he held a mirror to her mouth and detected a sign of moisture.

Forthwith he injected 6,000 milligrams of vitamin C, a staggering amount to put into the body of a one-and-one-half-year-old infant. Soon, however, the baby began to stir. In four hours she was alert, even cheerful, and was holding a bottle with her right hand. Her left side, however, remained paralyzed. Klenner then administered a second injection. Soon all signs of paralysis disappeared and the child, now laughing, could hold her bottle with two hands.

Klenner published the results of his work with vitamin C in the *Journal of Applied Nutrition* and in *Southern Medicine and Surgery* in the early 1950s. He has since gone on to become chief of staff at Reidsville Memorial Hospital, where he sees to it that nearly all extremely ill patients receive injections of 50,000 to 100,000 milligrams of vitamin C. Nevertheless, his work has gone largely unnoticed in the medical profession. The chances are that your own doctor has never heard of him.

This does not mean that other research into vitamin C has not gone forward. It has, and it is uncovering new possibilities in this simple vitamin all the time. Much of the research has taken place outside the United States. Thus, in Rumania the director of the Nutritional Research Center of the Institute of Medicine at Bucharest reported in 1968 that vitamin C reduced the toxicity of diphtheria, tetanus, and staph infections. At the Royal Children's Hospital in Australia, three doctors reported finding in 1974 that vitamin C helped make antibiotics more effective in treating a severe and stubborn germ (*Pseudomonas aeruginosa*), which tends to infect weakened hospital patients. The doctors' greatest surprise came, however, when they found that vitamin C could interact with drugs such as septrin, ampicillin, and erythromycin, which had, on their own, no effect on this bacterium, and turn these drugs into truly effective control agents.

In Singapore, a British dermatologist determined through a double-blind study in 1968 that vitamin C could combat prickly heat. In Czechoslovakia researchers giving vitamin C supplementation to miners to prevent colds found that the workers became more mentally alert at the same time. British scientist Roger Lewin told a 1974 medical conference in Britain of finding the same thing. (Dr. Klenner also believes that it boosts mental facility.)

In this country, James Greenwood, Jr., M.D., chief of neurosurgery at the Methodist Hospital in Houston, claims to have found vitamin C highly effective in eliminating many problems of the lower back. Dr. M. L. Riccitelli of the Yale School of Medicine apparently agrees, saying he has found the vitamin most useful in helping elderly patients with low back pain. Meanwhile another Yale team has discovered that vitamin C helps those who suffer from hay fever and other allergies. Finally, a rapidly rising accumulation of research indicates that vitamin C lowers cholesterol and helps prevent heart disease.

Can a vitamin that offers so much therapeutic value in the fight against so many human ailments play a role in the war against cancer? Some provocative and promising studies show that it can. Indeed, they suggest that it furnishes modern man with a major weapon for both preventing and treating this most dreaded of modern diseases. But before going on to examine these possibilities, let us first examine the biggest controversy that has engulfed this vitamin in recent years, namely its purported effect on the common cold. Such a study will shed valuable light not only on the potentialities of vitamin C, but also on the thought processes and therapeutic procedures that guide established medicine in modern America.

Vitamin C and the Common Cold

Not all the ailments and afflictions that Dr. Klenner found susceptible to vitamin C were major ones. The vitamin worked well in combating many minor illnesses as well. Like any other infection, Dr. Klenner found, the everyday cold tended to drain vitamin C from the human body. Or to put it another way, the human immunization system tended to consume vitamin C in combating cold germs. Consequently, Klenner recommended daily ingestion of vitamin C to help prevent colds and greatly increased dosages wherever the symptoms of a cold began to appear.

Nutritionist Adelle Davis and J. I. Rodale, publisher of *Prevention* magazine, heard about Klenner's findings, investigated, and became converts to his cause. They soon began to trumpet and tout the virtues of the vitamin as an antidote to colds. The medical community reacted largely with disinterest and disdain. After all, Davis was only a "pop lady nutritionist" with a simple master's degree while Rodale was an unsuccessful playwright who had become a "health nut." The fact that a bona fide physician had provided them with the basis for their belief was ignored.

However, evidence started to pour in from abroad attesting to the vitamin's efficacy in coping with colds. For example, on April 21, 1951, the *British Medical Journal* carried a letter from a husband-wife team of physicians, Doctors John M. and Isabel C. Fletcher, affirming vitamin C's ability to protect people against cold infection. The Doctors Fletcher expressed surprise that more research and reports had not been published about this. And in 1957 a Canadian ·physician, W. J. McCormick, of Toronto, was quoted as saying that he used vitamin C regularly in his practice to fight infections, including colds. Dr. McCormick urged people to start taking copious amounts of the vitamin as soon as the first signs of a cold appeared.

The real break in the issue came, however, in 1966, when biochemist Linus Pauling, winner of a Nobel prize in chemistry, found himself at an awards dinner sitting next to another biochemist named Irwin Stone. In the course of their dinner conversation, Pauling told Stone that there were many more things he would like to accomplish in life and so he would like to live another fifteen or twenty years. Stone subsequently sent off a regimen to Pauling calling for greatly increased ingestion of vitamin C. Pauling and his wife, who is a nutritionist herself, decided to follow the regimen. They both noticed that not only did they feel better, but they had begun to suffer from far fewer colds.

The welcome and somewhat unexpected effect that vitamin C produced on both him and his wife prompted Pauling to probe further. And in 1970 he published his book *Vitamin C and the Common Cold*. In it he stated that 2,000 units of vitamin C supplementation daily would protect most people most of the time from colds.

It was one thing for Davis and Rodale to sing hosannas to vitamin C; it was another thing for a well-known Nobel laureate to do so. (As one observer commented, "When Linus Pauling stops sneezing, it's not the same as when you and I stop sneezing.") Furthermore, Pauling, who has a rather ebullient personality anyway, had learned something about the use of publicity from his long extracurricular activities in the peace movement during the late forties and fifties. Soon he was causing the medical world to sit up and take notice.

Characteristically, the first research to test Pauling's thesis was done abroad. Two scientists at Trinity College in Dublin, Ireland, gave 500 milligrams of vitamin C to a group of school children. They found that the vitamin helped protect boys from colds, but did not seem to do as well in protecting girls. However, they concluded that consumption of 2,000 milligrams a day, Pauling's recommended dosage, "should provide resistance to the common cold in about 80% of teenage children."

In Scotland, meanwhile, a more careful study showed even more promising results. Doctors Sheila S. Charleston and K. Mary Clegg gave 1,000 milligrams of vitamin C daily to forty-seven people for a period of fifteen weeks. Another forty-three received a placebo. Writing in the *Lancet* on June 24, 1972, they reported that the group receiving vitamin C had suffered forty-four colds; the group receiving the placebo had experienced eighty colds, even though it was a somewhat smaller group. What's more, those colds that the vitamin C group caught did not, for the most part, last as long as those caught by the placebo takers.

The most thorough and best-regarded test, and one

that, for a while, started to turn the tide within the American medical profession itself, took place in Toronto. Dr. John Beaton, the head of the Department of Nutrition at the University of Toronto, had written a highly critical review of Pauling's book. Pauling had then fired off a letter to Beaton challenging him, in effect, to undertake a scientific test of his theory. Beaton had decided to pick up the gauntlet. He joined with two other doctors to carry out a most careful and controlled study that would, so they all assumed, put an end to Pauling, or at least to his claims about vitamin C.

Dr. Terrence W. Anderson actually headed the study. A noted epidemiologist, with a Ph.D. in addition to his medical degree, he too was hoping to disprove and debunk the vitamin C thesis. "Frankly," said Anderson afterwards, "when we began our study we intended to lay to rest all this business of megadoses of vitamin C. I didn't believe a word of Pauling's theory."

The researchers chose an especially large sample of 1,000 volunteers, of whom 818 stayed with the experiment to the end. Half were given 1,000 milligrams of vitamin C, the other half placebos. Great care was taken to keep the subjects from discovering which it was they were receiving, and a study afterwards showed that these efforts were successful. (Over two-thirds of both groups said they did not know whether they had received the vitamin C or the placebos. Of the remaining 32 percent who claimed they knew, half were right and half were wrong, indicating that they were only guessing.)

The results of the experiment are now well-known. The vitamin C takers lost 30 percent fewer days at work or school because of illness. Commented Dr. Anderson, "I was more than a little surprised when the results came out."

Anderson has since gone on to do two further studies of vitamin C, and each of them, he maintains, supports and strengthens the case for the vitamin. Indeed, he has found that it may actually have a greater effect on other illnesses than it does on the common cold. Writing in the *Canadian Medical Association Journal* of April 5, 1975, he noted, "There is now little doubt that the intake of additional vitamin C can lead to a reduced burden of winter illness." And he went on to say that "the effect observed was as great or even greater on illness not involving the nose."

By this time, some interest had started to stir in the United States. About a year after Anderson and his colleagues had reported the results of their vitamin C test, Dr. John E. Coulehan of the U.S. Public Health Service told a Stanford University symposium of an experiment he had conducted at a boarding school for Navajo children in Arizona. He gave half of the children in the six- to ten-year age group 1,000 milligrams a day, the other half received placebos. Half of the ten- to sixteen-year-olds, however, received 2,000 milligrams a day with the other half receiving placebos.

The results? The younger children given the vitamin C suffered 28 percent fewer sick days from colds than the control group. As for the older children who received the greater amount, they experienced 34 percent fewer sick days than their control group. Evidence was, thus, piling up to prove Pauling's point.

Overlooked heretofore in all controversy over vitamin C was the opinion of the physician who won the Nobel prize for discovering the vitamin in the 1930s, Albert Szent-Gyorgyi. *Prevention* magazine located the Hungarian-born researcher at Woods Hole, Massachusetts, where he was and is engaged in a branch of cancer research that we will be examining later on. Szent-Gyorgyi told the magazine that he had been taking at least 1,000 milligrams of the vitamin daily for some time and had found that it worked wonderfully in sparing him from the frequent colds that had plagued his younger years.

Meanwhile the growing evidence in vitamin C's behalf

was starting to score an impact on conventional American medicine. Reluctantly and, in many cases, almost remorsefully, physicians in the United States were beginning to back vitamin C as a preventive for colds. Said Washington cardiologist Dr. Patrick Gorman, "I read the [Pauling's] book, tried the pills, and they worked."

Dr. Gorman's statement appears in an article written by another Washington physician, internist Michael Halberstam, in the *New York Times Magazine* in 1974. The article provides some interesting and informative insight into how the modern medical mind reacts to research tending to support simple and nutritional therapeutic techniques.

"Ah, those were the days," Dr. Halberstam starts off, "those were the days when we doctors knew all about vitamins, and the people who stuffed themselves with B and C were cranks and food faddists, not Nobel prize winners!. . . we *knew* about vitamins then . . . we knew about vitamin supplements, too. We remembered the analogy from medical school about pouring extra coffee in a cup that was already filled—supplemental vitamins just sloshed over the brim, so to speak—coming out in the urine in amounts nearly proportional to the excessive intake. People took vitamins, we were told, because they did not understand nutrition and because advertising lured them with promises of greater strength and happiness. 'We have the richest urine in the world,' our medical school professors told us, and we laughed cynically."

"But," added Dr. Halberstam, "nobody's laughing now."

Halberstam went on to discuss some of the vitamin C studies concerning the common cold and noted, "There is quite simply mega-ignorance in the scientific community about megavitamins." The scientific journals, he said, appear "to have been overtaken by events during the current enthusiasm and physicians have little reliable information to fall back on. With the exception of an article reviewing vitamin E's action on the circulatory system, none of the major medical journals have published recent complete reviews of vitamin action and theory." And Halberstam pointed out that when the *New England Journal of Medicine* published Dr. Coulehan's article on his experiment in giving vitamin C to Navajo children, the *Journal* forsook its usual practice of commenting on the study. Said Halberstam, "I suspect that the journal's distinguished editorial board may have been so puzzled by the article that it couldn't agree as to what—if anything—the findings meant."

Halberstam himself was apparently still in the dark as to the wealth of research that existed on the other potentialities of vitamin C, research which, as we have seen, goes back to 1935. However, he did recount a meeting with a fellow internist who had gone to an orthopedist for a bad back. He was told by the specialist that he should try vitamin C. The internist told Halberstam, "I thought he was nuts with the vitamin C, but decided to give it a chance. It's crazy, but it works. When my back starts acting up, I take C and it goes away like magic. Don't ask me to explain it—*I'm embarrassed.*"

The words "I'm embarrassed" do not appear in italics in Dr. Halberstam's article, but I have added italics here for I believe these words offer us a valuable clue in understanding why modern medicine, especially American medicine, turns away from, and turns off to, the discoveries that their less conventional colleagues are making in nutritional research. The typical doctor does indeed find such research embarrassing. He also finds it somewhat threatening. For one thing, it does not jibe with what he learned in medical school. For another thing, if such simple remedies are available to an American doctor, then this will diminish the value of the strenuous efforts he made to acquire what is the most rigorous medical education in the world. Indeed, if nutrition can cure disease, then it may even, to some extent, put his livelihood in jeopardy. He does not want, in the words of the anti-Gerson doctor quoted in the previous chapter, "to chuck out millions of dollars of equipment in order to cook carrots in a pot."

Probably no doctor felt quite as threatened by the vitamin C controversy as did Dr. Frederick Stare. Dr. Stare teaches at the Harvard School of Medicine and directs its nutritional research activities. He has, thus, come to serve as the medical profession's foremost spokesman on nutritional matters. He has come to serve as the food industry's foremost spokesman as well, since he holds numerous contracts with major food processors. He once testified before a congressional subcommittee in behalf of sugared cereals.

For years, then, Stare has played the role of Horatius at the Bridge, defiantly and determinedly holding back the ignorant hordes of supernutritionists who threaten to sweep over his domain. Alarmed at the prestige and power which the supernutrition concept was gaining, thanks to Pauling's support, he took up the cudgels in behalf of traditional medicine.

He decided to focus his fire on Pauling and to disregard the fact that Szent-Gyorgyi was backing Pauling's claims. After all, Szent-Gyorgyi would be harder to discredit than Pauling, for he is even more greatly esteemed and his work in other areas is taught in medical schools. Since few people knew that Szent-Gyorgyi had endorsed the vitamin's anticold action, he could be safely omitted. (Of course, it is quite possible that Dr. Stare did not know Szent-Gyorgyi's opinion on the subject, although one would think that he would have checked with him before writing on the vitamin that Szent-Gyorgyi had discovered. The two men live only seventy miles from each other.)

In November 1969 Stare published an article in *Mademoiselle* in which he claimed that Pauling's claims about C were unfounded. If Pauling found himself getting fewer colds after taking vitamin C, then that resulted simply from the fact that Pauling was getting older, and older people get fewer colds. Stare also dredged up a 1942 study conducted at the University of Minnesota, which, he said, proved the uselessness of vitamin C in cold prevention. According to Stare, those who did the study took 5,000 students, divided them into two groups, gave one half "large doses" of vitamin C and the other half placebos. They found in two years of careful follow-up study that the vitamin C had made no difference in the "frequency, severity or duration of colds."

The contention that the relief from colds that Pauling and his wife experienced was a mere consequence of advancing age is scarcely convincing. Any such result would occur gradually over a period of time. The Paulings, however, had experienced relief right away. As for the Minnesota study, Pauling took a look at it himself and found, to his pleasant surprise, that it actually vindicated rather than vitiated his theory.

First of all, the Minnesota experiment involved only 400 students, not the 5,000 cited by Dr. Stare. Then, the "large dose" of vitamin C they received turned out to be 200 milligrams a day, or only one-tenth of what Pauling was recommending. Finally, and most importantly, even this small amount achieved a beneficial effect, for the vitamin C group suffered 15 percent fewer colds than the placebo group.

Pauling's repudiation of Stare, followed by the numerous previously cited studies showing positive results from vitamin C ingestion, seemed to be carrying the day for the vitamin C backers. However, the medical establishment was by no means ready to roll over and play dead. In 1974 the National Institute of Health (NIH) conducted a double-blind study of its own, and, wonder of wonders, its results revealed no significant effect of vitamin C on cold prevention. The *Journal of the American Medical Association* reported these results with evident relish in its March 10, 1975, issue. The medical traditionalists apparently felt they had finally rid themselves of vitamin C and the whole supernutrition fad. But let us take a look at the NIH experiment. The first thing we note is that it used a sample of 311. This was only about one-half the number used in the Navajo Indian experiment and not much more than one-third the number used by Dr. Anderson and his colleagues in their Toronto study. Now, any statistician will tell you that other things, being equal, the larger the sample, the more reliable the results. Anderson purposely chose a large sample because, as he said afterwards, "You need a large number of subjects to prove a negative." The NIH also wanted to prove a negative but did not choose to follow this advice.

A second factor that should strike our attention is the nature of the sample itself. It consisted entirely of NIH employees. This means that, to a great extent, it was made up of subjects who had almost a vested interest in disproving vitamin C's effectiveness. What's more, many of these subjects were medically sophisticated people who might easily be able to determine whether or not they were being given vitamin C or a placebo. (It will be recalled that although the doctors in the Toronto study were also hoping to disprove the vitamin C theory, they exercised the prudence of picking volunteers who had no stake in the outcome, and who had not been trained to recognize the taste of ascorbic acid or vitamin C. Furthermore, Anderson and his colleagues used a special filler with both the vitamin and the placebo to disguise any difference in taste. The NIH does not say that it took such precautionary measures.)

However, the most interesting result is that despite the prejudicial setting and the small sample, the experiment did show a slight variation between the two groups. The placebo takers averaged 1.36 colds apiece during the nine-month experimental period. The vitamin C takers averaged 1.27 colds—about 6 percent fewer colds.

All of these shortcomings notwithstanding, the American Medical Association seized on the study greedily, as a device to defend their traditional viewpoint. Indeed, one could almost hear a sigh of relief going up from the medical community. Many a doctor who had been wavering, now was able to return to the fold, secure in his belief that what he had been taught in medical school was true. There is something almost pathetic in the desperate way the leaders of medicine have used one flawed and faulty experiment to counteract the claims established by numerous, and much more thorough, studies. But such are the workings and the ways of so much modern medicine.

Vitamin C and Cancer

The Toronto study produced more than just proof that vitamin C can protect people from colds. It indicated that the vitamin's powers stretch into other areas as well. As a matter of fact, the vitamin C group enjoyed a 40 percent decrease in *all* illnesses, as compared to the control group, and this was greater than the decrease in colds alone. This fact caused Dr. Anderson and his colleagues to wonder whether vitamin C might have a general antiviral, antibacterial, antistress effect.

It stands to reason that any substance that might have such an effect, could have a role to play in fighting cancer. Meanwhile, several other research projects began to point to C's potentialities in the anticancer war.

Among these studies were two meticulous investigations carried out by doctors at the Medical Research Council in Cardiff, Wales. In one of these projects they closely examined the vitamin C intake in the diet of a group of nuns. In the other they surveyed the entire elderly population of a

Welsh village. They concluded that the vitamin C levels in a person's body, as measured by the concentration in their white cells, declined unmistakably with advancing years. Giving older persons supplementation of eighty milligrams a day would bring their vitamin C levels up to those of younger people, but it would take nine months for this to be accomplished. (They apparently did not experiment with the effect of larger amounts of supplementation. However, it is interesting to note that eighty milligrams a day is still more than double the recommended minimum amount from all sources that our own Public Health Service has prescribed.) Since cancer strikes the old more than the young, the study is at least suggestive.

Still more suggestive was a study done by an American physician, Dr. Emanuel Cheraskin. Dr. Cheraskin found that people with low levels of vitamin C in their blood tended to die at younger ages than those whose blood registered higher amounts of the vitamin. This finding underscores once again vitamin C's possible role in building and bolstering the body's immunization system. A later study found that people suffering from cancer almost invariably had low levels of vitamin C, oftentimes to the point of approaching scurvy.

Vitamin C research more closely connected to cancer was also emerging. For example, it was becoming apparent that a group of toxic chemicals called nitrites could cause cancer. It was not that they were carcinogenic in themselves, but that once introduced into the stomachs of laboratory animals, they would form what are called nitrosamines; nitrosamines are definitely carcenogenic. However, in 1972, four cancer specialists at the Eppley Institute for Research in Cancer at the University of Nebraska reported finding that vitamin C could, with sureness and speed, counteract this effect. If vitamin C was present in the stomach when the nitrites were introduced, no cancer-causing nitrosamines would ever be formed.

Chinese scientists made a similar finding when they set out to track down the cause of a minor cancer epidemic in a northwest province known as Linhsien. It seems that cancer of the esophagus (food pipe) was causing one out of every five deaths in the province. Investigation showed pickled cabbage, one of the province's favorite foods, to be the probable culprit. The pickling process produced nitrosamines. Furthermore, the Linhsienians preserved their pickled cabbage in earthenware jars that often became contaminated with a fungus. This fungus only enhanced the activity of the nitrosamines, adding to their potency and peril.

In examining a group of women from Linhsien, Chinese doctors found a high concentration of these nasty nitrosamines in their urine. However, after being given 900 milligrams a day of vitamin C, the nitrosamine content went down by 60 percent. The doctors suspended the vitamin supplementation to see what would happen. Sure enough, in three days the nitrosamines began to increase noticeably.

If vitamin C can destroy at least some of the substances that cause cancer, can it destroy cancer itself? Evidence of its effectiveness in controlling and even curing one form of the disease emerged from Tulane University in 1968. Dr. J. U. Schlegal, a urologist at Tulane's medical school, reported on some research carried out by himself and three colleagues from the school's Department of Surgery. They implanted a proven bladder carcinogen in mice and then added vitamin C to their drinking water. The result? The mice did not develop cancer.

Dr. Schlegal then began administering vitamin C to patients suffering from bladder cancer. Bladder cancer, it should be pointed out, is one of the more formidable forms of the disease. Some twenty-five thousand Americans develop it every year, and over ten thousand of them will die as a result. However, Schlegal found that when his patients took 1,500 milligrams a day of vitamin C, they almost always survived.

Gratifying as this news was, it still only affects 3 percent of all cancer cases. What about the other 97 percent who suffer cancer in other parts of the body? An observation made by both Pauling and Cheraskin provides food for thought. They both called attention to the fact that vitamin C is not uniformly distributed throughout the body. Some organs contain a good deal of vitamin C; some contain very little. Cancer also does not strike all organs of the body with uniform frequency. Some organs are much less likely to become cancerous than others. The organs that contain the most vitamin C are the most likely to escape the disease. For example, the vitamin C content of the adrenal gland is very high; ergo, cancer of the adrenal gland is very rare.

In the face of these snowballing studies suggesting vitamin C's potential for curbing cancer, sentiment began to build up for a more all-embracing attempt to determine vitamin C's ability to defeat the disease. The stage was being set for the Glasgow experiment.

Putting Vitamin C to the Test

In the early 1970s two Scottish physicians from the Glasgow area, Doctors Evan Cameron and Allan Campbell, had become impressed with the increasing indications that vitamin C improves the body's mechanism for defending itself against infection and attack. They had observed that laboratory animals who were able to manufacture their own vitamin C produced greatly increased amounts of it when injected with a cancer-causing chemical (methylcholanthrene). Rats, for example, would generate the equivalent for an average-sized human being of 16,000 milligrams a day.

The two doctors selected fifty cancer patients whom two independent physicians certified as being beyond medical aid. They administered to them 2,500 milligrams of C four times a day—or 10,000 milligrams daily—and closely observed the results.

Some seventeen, or about one-third of the patients, showed no improvement at all. Ten other patients registered what the Scottish doctors called a "minimal response." This means that they showed some immediate improvement, but it failed to last. In another eleven patients, the growth of cancer definitely slowed down, though it did not stop. For example, a sixty-seven-year-old man with advanced cancer of the gall bladder and liver, who was not expected to last the month, found his appetite returning after a week on vitamin C. He began to gain weight and was able to return home, where he died seven months after starting the vitamin C treatment.

In eight of the patients, meanwhile, the growth of cancer came to a full stop and in some cases even regressed. In three of them the disease eventually resumed its progress and, eventually, took their lives. One lived almost two more years before succumbing. Two others died from other causes, and autopsies performed on their bodies showed that their cancer had significantly subsided. Finally, three, at last report, were still alive and functioning normally.

Of course, cancer, even in its terminal stages, very occasionally takes a temporary turn for the better. On even rarer occasions it clears up. But, say Doctors Campbell and Cameron, "It is our opinion that most clinicians familiar with the practical realities of terminal cancer . . . would tend to agree that many of these patients survived much longer than reasonable clinical expectation."

However, if you have been keeping count you will notice that four of the fifty patients remain unaccounted for. What happened to them? These patients, so it seems, suffered fatal hemorrhages as a result of the vitamin C. Does this mean that vitamin C can prove dangerous to cancer sufferers and, therefore, should be avoided? The Scottish doctors feel just the opposite. They regarded this seemingly negative reaction on the part of 8 percent of the patients as actually further proof of vitamin C's ability to attack cancer. It seems that the fatal hemorrhages resulted from the fact that the vitamin C destroyed their tumors. However, the tumors were already so large that the effect proved fatal. Thus, the doctors regarded this as "a manifestation of the very strong defense reaction" engendered by the vitamin C. Such a reaction "would certainly be regarded as a favorable response, indeed, in patients suffering from earlier and more localized" forms of the disease.

The experiment produced several other positive consequences. One patient who had a problem with jaundice found this ailment improving. Some were suffering from a malignant disease of the urinary tract. The blood in their urine decreased markedly. Their pain and distress also eased. As a matter of fact, nearly all the patients felt better, including most of the seventeen who showed no other positive response. Five patients had required continuous large doses of morphine to alleviate their agony. All of them were able to be taken off the drug without suffering any increased pain or even any withdrawal symptoms.

What about side effects? The doctors had wondered if such heavy dosages might not develop kidney stones, but none of the fifty patients experienced such a problem. A few, especially those suffering from cancer in the upper alimentary tract, did experience nausea and acid regurgitation (heartburn) from the vitamin. But that was all.

For those who still might remain unconvinced of the experiment's evidence regarding the anticancer properties of vitamin C, the researchers cite the case of one of the patients who survived. He was a forty-two-year-old truck driver who had been admitted to the hospital with cancer in a widespread network of organs and tissues known as the RE system. (It includes blood and lymph vessels, bone marrow, spleen, lymph nodes, and liver.)

After ten days on vitamin C the afflicted man's liver and spleen had shrunk to normal size. The diseased condition of his lymph nodes was rapidly improving. His appetite returned, his night sweats stopped, and he said he felt quite well. In January 1974, after three months in the hospital, his chest X ray was normal, and he was able to return to work.

As he continued to thrive, the doctors tapered off the vitamin C dosages, and by the end of March they ended them completely. But, after four weeks without the vitamin supplementation, patient 45, as he was called, began experiencing cancer symptoms. His cough and weariness returned. Readmitted to the hospital, his chest X rays showed enlargement of the tissues between the lungs.

The physicians hastily resumed the vitamin C treatment, but this time it did not seem to help. In a final effort to bring the malignancy under control, they doubled the dose. For two weeks he received 20,000 milligrams a day. Then they reduced it to 12,500 milligrams a day, which still came to 25 percent more than the original amount.

More gradually than before, he began to improve. By November 1974 his chest X ray was again back to normal. He is now back at work but continues to take 12,500 milligrams every day.

Heartened by results such as these, the two Scottish physicians decided to push forward to gather more evidence. They selected another group of fifty cancer victims, each of whom had been examined by at least two other doctors and had been judged to be beyond any medical aid. These patients also received 10,000 milligram doses of the vitamin daily, and they responded in the same way as the first group. Meanwhile, the two physicians went through their hospital's records until they found at least ten cases comparable in type of cancer, age, sex, and so on to every one of the 100 they had not treated with vitamin C. They then evaluated what happened to each vitamin C recipient as compared to what happened to the ten cases used as controls. (These "controls" were now dead. However, their records were used to make the comparison.)

By this time Linus Pauling and his institute had become associated with the experiment, and in October 1976 Pauling and one of the Scottish physicians, Evan Cameron, published a paper in the *Proceedings of the National Academy of Sciences*. Their report startled the medical community, or at least startled all those in the medical community who bothered to read it.

The 1,000 patients whose medical records had served as controls had lived, on the average, for 50.4 days. The 100 patients who received the vitamin C had lived, on the average, 209.6 days. *Thus the survival rate of the vitamin C recipients was more than four times greater than that of the others!*

The increased survival rates showed up in virtually all the various cancer categories. The stomach cancer patients, for example, lived nearly 2.67 times longer than their "controls." Those with lung cancer survived, on the average, over 3.50 times longer. Bladder cancer patients remained alive 4.50 times longer, breast cancer patients 5.75 times longer and colon cancer sufferers 7.61 times longer than those who had never received the vitamin C.

Refining the figures still more, Pauling and Cameron pointed out that 90 percent of the vitamin C–treated patients lived only about three times as long as the control patients but 10 percent of them lived at least *twenty times as long*. As a matter of fact many of them were still alive with their cancer apparently under control.

If vitamin C wars against cancer, then how does it do so? Pauling believes that it does so in two ways. First, it increases the formation of what is known as collagen. And collagen acts as as the cement that holds the tissue together. By strengthening collagen in the tissues, vitamin C may make the tissues more cancer-resistant. Secondly, says Pauling, vitamin C steps up the production of lymphocytes, which serve as one of the chief defenders against illness.

Robert Yonemoto, M.D., who directs the surgical laboratories at the City of Hope National Medical Center at Duarte, California, apparently agrees with Pauling on this point. Dr. Yonemoto told *Prevention* that giving patients 5,000 milligrams of vitamin C daily increased their lymphocyte production. When he doubled the dose to 10,000 milligrams a day, the lymphocyte production went up still more. "Vitamin C increases the general immunity of the individual," said the California surgeon.

Gradually, the idea that vitamin C can help and help greatly in keeping a person cancer-free is gaining ground. For example, Dr. Paul Chretien, chief of tumor immunology for the National Cancer Institute, has admitted that vitamin C stimulates the body's defense system "and this usually means an increased immune response."[1] Nevertheless, at this

---

[1]Dr. Chretien's remarks were made in response to a query from the Associated Press in October 1976. (The news service's interest was probably provoked by the Pauling-Cameron report in the *Proceedings* of the same month.) *Nature's Way* magazine followed up Dr. Chretien's statement by seeking the data on which it was based. Securing the data, said the magazine in its June 1977 issue, proved no easy task. Yet, eventually it learned that the institute had given 5,000 to 10,000 milligrams of vitamin C a day to five healthy volunteers and had observed that the intake appeared to improve the ability of the subjects' white blood cells to fight infection.

Probing further, *Nature's Way* came across a 1969 report in the scientific journal *Oncology* that revealed some interesting laboratory work by institute biochemists. The scientists found vitamin C to be highly lethal to cancer cells when placed with the latter in a test tube. Yet the vitamin remained remarkably nontoxic to normal body tissues. The researchers also found that test animals could absorb more than 2,000 milligrams of vitamin C *for each pound of body weight* without any observable deleterious effects. If true for man, this would mean that a 150-pound person could ingest well over 300,000 milligrams a day without harm.

writing most doctors are still rejecting or ignoring the mounting pile of solid, substantial evidence that is accumulating in vitamin C's behalf.

The real tragedy is that this evidence goes back not just to the Glasgow experiment but much further. In his 1971 book *The Healing Factor*, Dr. Irwin Stone devotes a chapter to reviewing all the research on vitamin C and cancer that had up to then been published. We find expe.iments showing its anticancer effect being reported as far back as the 1940s. One case, which appeared in the *Medical Times* in 1954, is of particular interest for it deals with dosages substantially larger than even those used in the Glasgow experiment.

As written up by the attending physician, it concerns the case of a seventy-three-year-old business executive who was suffering from a multitude of medical problems including alcoholic cirrhosis of the liver. On top of all this he developed chronic leukemia, or cancer of the blood.

On his own initiative, the patient started taking *24,500 to 42,000 milligrams of vitamin C a day*, claiming he felt much better when he took such gargantuan dosages. He even returned to his job with a major oil company. Twice, at the insistence of his alarmed physician, he stopped taking such megadoses of the vitamin. Each time he did so, his spleen and liver enlarged and became tender, his temperature rose to 101 degrees Fahrenheit, and he complained of general malaise and fatigue, which are typical leukemia symptoms. But when he resumed his vitamin C consumption, the symptoms cleared and his temperature became normal *within six hours*.

The man died in a year and a half from other medical problems. But at the time of death *neither the leukemia nor the cirrhosis had shown any sign of progression*. As the apparently somewhat bewildered physician concluded, "The intake of the huge doses of ascorbic acid [vitamin C] appeared essential for the welfare of the patient."

Stone, in reporting the case, properly bewails the fact

that none of the groups dedicated to fighting leukemia have ever bothered to make use of it, even as a basis for further study. If extremely high vitamin C absorption "could do so much for an aged leukemic with so many other complications," says Dr. Stone, "what could it do for the young, uncomplicated leukemic?"

It may be one of the major tragedies of modern medicine that Stone's question is still awaiting an answer.

Vitamin C: How Much Is Enough?

If we go back and look once again at the Gerson diet, we will find that it contained fairly generous amounts of vitamin C. The raw vegetable and fruit juices, which were the mainstay of Dr. Gerson's regimen, should have provided the patient with a much greater intake of the vitamin than he would otherwise have consumed. Today, with the work of Klenner, Pauling, Schlegal, Cheraskin, Cameron, Campbell, and others to guide us, we can see that still more vitamin C may be necessary to protect and preserve us from cancer.

Before trying to determine a desirable dosage, however, let us first take a look at what may be the reason that man needs to obtain vitamin C from an outside source. You will recall that most animals manufacture their own vitamin C. Man and other primates are some of the very few exceptions. Dr. Irwin Stone, in his above-cited book, outlines a theory as to why this is so.

According to Stone, early man, or one of his evolutionary forebears, originally possessed the capacity to generate the vitamin within his own body. However, a genetic malfunctioning occurred, at least partly from the fact that he was obtaining all the vitamin C he needed from his diet. At that time this diet consisted basically of raw fruits and vegetables. No longer needing to make his own vitamin C, he eventually lost his ability to do so. But man's diet has changed since then, and today he consumes relatively few foods containing substantial amounts of vitamin C. The normal human diet of today, even if it includes a glass of orange juice for breakfast and salads at both lunch and dinner will still, according to the Stone theory, fail by a wide margin to provide sufficient quantities of vitamin C for optimum health.

Pauling, among others, has associated himself with Stone's theory. The Nobel laureate points out that if modern man obtained 2,500 calories a day from raw and natural plant food as his predecessors presumably did, he would also be obtaining about 2,300 milligrams of vitamin C. This, says Pauling, is about forty-two times the amount of vitamin C currently recommended for a person whose daily energy requirement comes to 2,500 calories.

Two other factors should also be kept in mind. Though the evidence suggests that vitamin C possesses great power, it also shows that it is quite fragile. It is easily destroyed in food through cooking and is easily erased in the human body through smoking as well as through stress, including not just the physical stress of an infection or illness, but emotional stress as well. Finally, vitamin C is virtually nontoxic, and there are no reports of a serious illness, let alone a death, resulting from too much vitamin C ingestion. Sodium chloride, or salt, is much more toxic, and yet the average American, according to nutritionist Jean Mayer, consumes daily about ten times as much as he needs.

With all these points in mind, how much extra vitamin C should we take every day to guard us from cancer and to give us the maximum benefits that the vitamin can bestow?

Dr. Klenner takes 20,000 milligrams a day and claims all adults should take at least 10,000 a day. Children under the age of ten, he says, should receive 1,000 milligrams a day for each year of life. Such an intake, says this physician, will, in addition to preventing much illness, cause the individual to find that "the brain will be clearer, the mind more active, the body less wearied, and the memory more retentive."

Dr. Pauling, at last report, was taking 6,000 milligrams a day but was thinking of increasing his consumption to Klenner's recommended dosage. Dr. Szent-Gyorgyi contents himself with consuming 1,000 to 2,000 milligrams a day. It is interesting to observe that Dr. Klenner is already past seventy, Dr. Pauling is nearly eighty, while Dr. Szent-Gyorgyi is into his mid-eighties. All three men follow extremely busy and productive schedules and none of them has sustained a major illness.[2]

However, if one still has qualms about the need and desirability of taking vitamin C supplementation, and has fears as to its consequences, then further assurance is available from Dr. Charles E. Butterworth, Jr., a member of the editorial board of the *Journal of the American Medical Association* and former chairman of the AMA's Food and Nutrition Council. Dr. Butterworth feels that 1,000 to 2,000 milligrams of vitamin C may represent the ideal daily ration.

Butterworth made this suggestion in 1974 after reviewing research showing that vitamin C could lower cholesterol and help protect the heart. Except for a general statement made earlier, no attempt has been made to report on this research here, for it does not seem sufficiently connected with cancer prevention and treatment to warrant our attention. But the fact that it has impressed one of the most respected members of the AMA's hierarchy opens up hope for the future. Perhaps, some day, your own doctor will nod

---

[2]Nutritionist Adelle Davis did die of cancer at the age of seventy. However, she only believed in taking vitamin C supplements in cases of colds or other infections. Furthermore, as we will see in a later chapter, her dietary recommendations include some substances that tend to promote cancer.

approvingly instead of smiling scornfully when you tell him or her that you take 2,000 milligrams of vitamin C a day. Maybe someday your doctor will even recommend it to you.

But none of us can afford to await such a memorable or momentous event. We should all be taking generous amounts of the vitamin now, for it alone may keep us cancer-free. And if it proves insufficient by itself to protect us completely from cancer, then do not despair. Many more nutritional weapons are coming to the fore to help us win the anticancer war.

4

The A B E's of Cancer Prevention

Vitamin C may play a crucial, even cardinal, role in helping us resist cancer. But it need not, indeed should not, fight alone. Many other vitamins have also demonstrated a capacity to curb and constrain this malignancy. As we shall now see, they can become valuable allies in our anticancer program.

Vitamin A

In 1955, the *Journal of Nutrition* published some pioneering and provocative research by two Chicago scientists. B. M. Kagan of Michael Reese Hospital and Elizabeth Kaiser of Northwestern University Medical School had found that children suffering from rheumatic fever showed low blood levels of vitamin A. They noticed the same effect in pneumonia patients. In fact, as they investigated further, they discovered that any fever seemed to decrease sharply the amount of vitamin A in the body.

They then proceeded to induce inflammations in laboratory rats with the aim of producing something similar to a bacterial abscess. Sure enough, such stressful situations caused their blood and liver levels of the vitamin to drop sharply. Here was evidence, as we have already seen with vitamin C, that a vitamin was being utilized and used up to ward off an attack.

Some twelve years later, a London physician, Dr. Max Odens, told of his experiences in giving vitamin A to patients suffering from chronic bronchitis. He had begun administering the vitamin, along with the usual therapy, to some seventeen patients in the early 1950s. At the time he wrote his article, some fifteen years later, all of them were still alive, with the eldest being seventy-nine. Furthermore, all of them, said Dr. Odens, had shown considerable improvement. (His article appeared in the German medical publication *Vitalstoffe* in December, 1967.)

Skipping ahead five years we find a Phoenix, Arizona, surgeon, Dr. Merrill Chernov, telling his colleagues that surgical stress consumes large amounts of vitamin A. Writing in the *American Journal of Surgery,* Dr. Chernov claimed that the best way to treat such stress was to give the patient large dosages of vitamin A. He noted that he administered as much as 100,000 international units of vitamin A after major surgery.

In 1973 another surgeon, Dr. Benjamin E. Cohen of Massachusetts General Hospital, told a meeting of the American Society of Plastic and Reconstructive Surgeons, that vitamin A strengthens the ability of laboratory animals to fight off infection. He reported how he had inoculated mice with 3,000 units of vitamin A, an enormous amount for such a tiny animal. He had then injected the mice with deadly bacteria. Another group of mice that had not been given the vitamin A also received the bacteria.

The non–vitamin A recipients all died of infection after twenty-four hours. The mice that had received the vitamin developed severe infections for the first three hours. But at the end of five hours, the infections seemed to have disappeared. As Dr. Cohen put it, "No more [bacteria] organisms could be cultured from their blood."

In testing out other forms of infectious bacteria against vitamin-A-inoculated animals, Dr. Cohen had found the responses to be similar. To be sure, many of the animals had succumbed to some types of the bacteria with which he inoculated them. But in all cases those animals fortified with greatly increased amounts of vitamin A resisted the infections much better.

Resisting bacteria is one thing; resisting a virus is another. However, in 1975 a professor of biochemistry and surgery at the Albert Einstein College of Medicine reported success with vitamin A in this area as well. Dr. Eli Seifter told a meeting of the American Chemical Society that he had injected pox virus into two groups of mice. One group had been given five to ten times its usual daily requirement of vitamin A. The other had received the normal amount present in the usual laboratory diet. The results? The vitamin A–fed mice developed fewer pox lesions, and those they did develop cleared up faster than did those that the control animals developed. Furthermore the mice that received the vitamin suffered less fever than did the mice that served as controls.

Dr. Seifter drew from his experiments the conclusion that vitamin A is "very protective" and enhances the body's ability to immunize itself against attack. His finding and his experiments, along with the other experiments and findings we have examined, seem, in many ways, to parallel those that we examined in the previous chapter on vitamin C. This is by no means a coincidence, for vitamin A does appear to produce some of the effects of vitamin C. Like its more recently discovered rival, vitamin A does seem to do its good work not in directly fighting illness itself but in helping the body's own immunization system do its job.

All of this would seem to indicate that vitamin A might have a stellar part to play in the anticancer drama. And so it does. Indeed, in some respects, it may rival, if not surpass, that of vitamin C in helping to keep us cancer-free.

Research into the relationship between vitamin A and cancer actually goes back to 1942. It was in that year that Dr. I. S. Tannock and his co-workers from the Anderson Hospital and Tumor Institute of the University of Texas at Houston first reported on the results of administering the vitamin to an animal that was being given radiation treatment for a tumor. They claimed such vitamin A ingestion reduced the amount of radiation needed to control the tumor by 25 percent. The more time the animal had to absorb and assimilate the vitamin, the better it was able to handle the tumor.

Like so much of the early research done by Jungeblut in vitamin C, this research remained largely ignored for many years. However, in a 1967 article covering the use of vitamin A in aiding chronic bronchitis, Dr. Odens also disclosed some results of his use of the vitamin in cancer control. He found that cancer-causing substances applied to the neck of the uterus would not cause cervical cancer if vitamin A were added to them. He noted that although cancer cultured outside the body could be induced into prostate glands, this did not occur when the carcinogen used to induce the cancer was supplemented with vitamin A.

The real break in the vitamin A cancer story did not occur, however, until the following year when Dr. Umberto Saffioti, then a pathologist at Chicago Medical School, related some of his research results to a conference at MIT. Dr. Saffiotti told of exposing 113 hamsters to high dosages of benzypyrene, a known carcinogen found in tobacco smoke. Some 60 of the animals had previously been given substantial amounts of vitamin A. The other 53 had not. Of the 53 animals that had not received the vitamin, 16 developed lung cancer. *Of the 60 animals that had received the vitamin, only 1 developed any cancerous tumors.*

Vitamin A's benefits were not confined solely to the lungs. Further experiments, said Dr. Saffiotti, showed that it also tended to protect the forestomach, the gastrointestinal tract, and the uterine cervix from cancer. He said that other laboratory animals had also been tested with vitamin A and had been found to have achieved substantial protection against malignancy, thanks to the vitamin.

The Saffiotti report spurred numerous medical researchers to experiment with vitamin A. The result has been a steady stream of reported research in the seventies, all of it favorable. In 1971 Dr. Raymond J. Shamberger of the Cleveland Clinic Foundation, reported on a series of experiments with mice, rabbits, and hamsters. He flatly concluded that "vitamin A, when administered topically or systemically [externally or internally], retards the growth and inhibits the induction of benign and malignant tumors."

Two years later, a team of researchers from the Albert Einstein College of Medicine told a conference at Cornell University of finding not only that vitamin A seemed to protect mice from induced tumors, but that when such vitamin-protected mice did develop malignancy, their tumors developed much more slowly than they did with non-vitamin-protected mice and regressed about twice as fast.

Similar research has also been reported from Vanderbilt University, the National Cancer Institute, the National Institute of Allergy and Infectious Diseases, and MIT. In all cases, vitamin A was found to inhibit the growth of cancer.

However, all these investigations dealt solely with laboratory animals. What is still lacking at the time of this writing is something comparable to the Edinborough experiment wtih vitamin C, which was discussed in the previous chapter. So far, no one has published any research on the administration of vitamin A to human cancer sufferers.

We do, however, have a report from Norway that indicates, as is so often the case, that what works for laboratory animals can also work for humans. In 1975, Dr. E. Bjelke of the Cancer Registry of Norway, disclosed the results of a five-year study involving 8,278 men. Dr. Bjelke classified the men into two groups, those whose vitamin A intake was low and those whose vitamin A intake was *relatively* high. His classification does not mean that the latter were taking extra amounts of the vitamin, but only that their regular diet gave them somewhat more vitamin A than the low–vitamin A group.

What did he find? Well, although only one-third of the total number of men fell into the low–vitamin A group, *that group was responsible for nearly three-quarters of all the lung cancer in both groups combined.* Put another way, those whose diet gave them less of the vitamin had more than three times the chance of developing lung cancer than those whose diet was somewhat better supplied. The statistical discrepancy between the two groups is sufficiently sizable to suggest that vitamin A can help, and help mightily, in the war against cancer.

Another statistical correlation may also be of some relevance in this regard. The steady upward swing in the American cancer rate—cancer deaths increased more than 4 percent in 1975 over 1974—has been accompanied by a slow, but steady, decline of vitamin A in the American diet. It has been estimated that in 1950, the average American ate thirty-one pounds more of fresh fruits and twenty pounds more of fresh vegetables than he did in 1970. Taking the place of the missing fruits and vegetables in the American diet were beef, pork, and junk foods of various kinds, none of which contain appreciable amounts of vitamin A.

Several studies done in the early seventies bear out this falloff in vitamin A intake and show its dimensions. For example, autopsies performed on 372 bodies in various parts of the nation indicated that up to 37 percent of them were deficient in the vitamin. These people had come from various income groups and had died from various causes. Yet, the pattern of deficiency touched all the groups equally. Elderly women seem to be particularly prone to be lacking this vitamin. A ten-state survey completed under the aegis of the U.S. Department of Health, Education, and Welfare in 1970 showed that fully 68.5 percent of women over sixty were not getting their recommended daily allowances of vitamin A. As a matter of fact, two out of five women were not even getting 2,000 units a day, which is only 40 percent of the 5,000 units recommended. And the research already noted suggests that adequate cancer protection requires much greater amounts than the RDA figure of 5,000 units.

How much vitamin A is required for adequate cancer protection? What foods best supply it? Is there a difference in the kinds of vitamin A available in tablet form? How much is too much? These and other matters will be examined later on when we will attempt to draw up an anticancer regimen. In the meantime, however, anyone concerned about cancer should put vitamin A next to vitamin C on his weapon list.

The B Vitamins

In the early 1940s, medical workers at the New York Skin and Cancer Hospital were looking for a better way to treat *precancerous* lesions in the soft tissues of the month. They were struck by one fact. These lesions strongly resembled those that appear in people suffering from pellagra. Why not, they wondered, try to treat the lesions as if they were pellagra? They decided to do so. They gave the patients a diet high in the B complex vitamins along with stepped-up amounts of protein. Lo and behold, the precancerous lesions disappeared.

Some years later, two researchers at a Canadian medical school compared a group of women suffering from cancer of the reproductive tract with a group of cancer-free women of the same age. They were struck by the fact that nearly 95 percent of the women who had cancer also had an elevated output of female hormone and a low level of B complex vitamins. Their diets were low in the B vitamins as well as in protein. The cancer-free women, according to Dr. Carlton Fredericks, "showed a diametrically opposite picture: normal or low output of female hormone, diets well supplied with vitamin B complex and protein, and therefore blood levels within normal range." Fredericks claims that this study and the previously related incident from the New York Skin and Cancer Hospital, show the effect of diet on cancer. It may be inferred, from these examples, that the B vitamins have a role to play in combatting cancer.

One of the best sources of the B vitamins is brewers yeast. Another good source is liver. These facts may figure into an intriguing case study reported in the *American Journal of Surgery* of August 1942.

Two physicians had administered on a daily basis three tablespoons of brewers yeast plus liver to a man suffering from cancer of the mouth. The patient soon regained twenty-five pounds and his malignancy seemed to have regressed. Then, one and a half years later, his cancer once again began to gain ground. His daily intake of brewers yeast was now boosted to eight tablespoons a day, which is a lot of brewer's yeast. Again his cancer appeared to come under control. And as long as he continued on his brewers yeast regimen, he continued to feel well.

It was quite possibly this case that inspired Dr. Kanematsu Sugiura to conduct a rather remarkable experiment some eight years later. Dr. Sugiura, a Japanese-American biochemist employed by the Sloan-Kettering Institute of Cancer Research, had come across a chemical that would give laboratory animals liver cancer in about 150 days. He fed the carcinogen to four different groups of rats.

As reported in the July 10, 1951, *Journal of Nutrition*, the first group received the cancer-causing chemical along with a regular rat diet. The second group, however, received a supplement of brewer's yeast amounting to 3 percent of their dietary intake. The amount of the yeast was raised to 6 percent for the third group and to 15 percent for the fourth group. Dr. Sugiura then waited to see if the yeast would delay or deter the onslaught of cancer.

As expected, the fifty animals that received the regular diet all developed cancer of the liver in about 150 days. At this time none of the rats receiving the supplements of brewer's yeast showed any sign of cancer. Later, some of them did develop malignancy, but the differences in degree revealed some interesting information. Of the group receiving 3 percent brewer's yeast in their diets, 30 percent remained cancer-free. Of the group receiving 6 percent brewer's yeast 70 percent remained cancer-free. And of the group that received 15 percent brewer's yeast, none showed any sign of liver cancer whatsoever!

Although the experiment disclosed that brewer's yeast seemed to display a surprising capacity to curb cancer, the conclusions to be drawn from it in terms of the B vitamins remain more complex. Brewer's yeast also contains many other substances, including a trace mineral that more recent research has shown to be a strong inhibitor. (We will examine this mineral in the next chapter.) Furthermore, the B complex is itself quite complex. It consists of vitamins B_1, B_2, B_3, B_6, and B_{12}, as well as choline, inositol, biotin, folic acid, pantothenic acid, and para-aminobenzoic acid. Some other vitamin B substances might be included as well. To the extent that the B vitamins tend to prevent cancer, do they act as a group or individually? In other words, is it only some of the B vitamins that are enemies of cancer, or is it all of them?

At this stage there appears to be no satisfactory answer to this question. In 1943 the magazine *Science* reported that injections of inositol slowed down the growth of transplanted tumors. Five years later, the *Journal of Urology* carried a report of how inositol, given to six bladder cancer patients, reduced the size of their tumors and stopped blood from appearing in their urine.

Dr. Roger J. Williams, probably the country's most outstanding researcher in the area of nutrition, calls attention to several experiments that showed how a deficiency in choline produced cancer in rats. However, in his highly regarded book, *Nutrition Against Disease*, Dr. Williams cautions against drawing too much from these experiments. While choline may be the "limiting factor" in rats, this does not mean that it plays the same role in man.

A Canadian urologist, Dr. Balfour M. Mount of the Royal Victoria Hospital and McGill University, says he has found vitamin B_6 to be effective in helping bladder cancer victims. It does this, says Dr. Mount, by normalizing the patient's metabolism of tryptophane. (Tryptophane is one of the protein-building amino acids.) He feels that a daily intake of 200 milligrams of this B vitamin "may rectify the whole metabolic picture where some cancer-causing chemicals are concerned."

Some particularly promising research came to light in 1972 when the findings of a six-member team from the University of California at Los Angeles and the Nucleic Acid Research Institute of Irvine, California, were published. The researchers found that cancer cells consistently lacked vita-min B_3, sometimes called niacinamide. Normal cells, on the other hand, consistently contained this B vitamin. Further-more, adding niacinamide or B_3 to laboratory cultures of cancer cells inhibited the abnormal protein synthesis that seems to characterize cancer cells.

These experiments were exciting, but they were, as yet, confined to the test tube. Researchers must still try out the effects of B_3 on humans or even laboratory animals. Further investigation may show B_3 to be a strong, and even decisive, anticancer agent; the returns are not yet in.

Another member of the B family, para-aminobenzoic acid, has been found to be extremely effective in warding off the most common form of cancer, skin cancer. Skin cancer is the least deadly form of cancer and, therefore, is not greatly feared. Nevertheless, of the 300,000 people who contract it every year, 5,000 will die as a result. Consequently, despite its low mortality rate, it is not to be taken lightly.

Three Harvard Medical School dermatologists have found para-aminobenzoic acid, or PABA as it is sometimes called, more effective than all commercially available prod-ucts in protecting fair-skinned persons against long exposure to the sun (such exposure is the primary cause of skin cancer). In 1969 they tested twenty-four suntan lotions, along with three different solutions of PABA, on people in the Arizona desert and high in the Swiss Alps. The PABA uniformly came through with flying colors.

Viewing the cancer problem from the more general perspective of building up the human body's overall im-munization ability, we find that several members of the B complex family come into play. However, there is some dis-agreement among the experts as to which are the most im-portant. For Dr. A. E. Axelrod of Pittsburgh University Med-ical School, B_6, folic acid, and pantothenic acid are the crucial crusaders in the immunization process. He told a seminar on

Nutrition and the Future of Man in 1971 that no animal can produce sufficient antibodies to protect itself from disease if these B vitamins are missing. In some cases, said Dr. Axelrod, "no circulatory antibodies whatsoever can be produced in the absence of these specific factors."

Dr. Paul Newberne, a researcher in nutritional pathology at MIT, includes folic acid on his list of four specific nutrients, which he says do yeoman work in protecting us from disease. However, in place of pantothenic acid and B_6, he substitutes choline and B_{12}. (The fourth and final nutrient on his list is methionine, an essential amino acid used to build protein.)

Finally, Dr. Otto Warburg, winner of two Novel prizes, singled out in 1966 three B vitamins as powerful and potent cancer fighters. These are B_2, B_3, and pantothenic acid. These three B vitamins, said the distinguished doctor, played the most vital role in manufacturing the critical enzymes needed to regulate the metabolic processes in order to protect people from malignancy.

To sum up, the role of the B vitamins in the wide-ranging war against cancer remains complicated indeed. The research, as yet, is far from complete and far from clear. What is apparent, however, is that at least some of the B vitamins do possess anticancer properties. Although we do not yet know with certainty which ones they are, that should not greatly concern us. Fortunately, the best sources of this complex clan of nutrients contain them all. These sources include brewer's yeast, liver, and wheat germ. In addition, tablets that contain them all are readily available.

Our best bet, then, is simply to include the B complex in its entirety on our anticancer agenda. Indeed, there is actually some danger in taking too much of any one B vitamin, for that can, in some instances, lead to a deficiency in some of the others. Therefore, taking them all may well protect us from other problems as well.

Vitamin E

Vitamin E has become a fashionable vitamin in recent years, much too fashionable in the eyes of establishment medicine. While everyone accepts the fact that the vitamin is needed in human nutrition, many deplore the exaggerated claims that have been made in its behalf. One medical publication, *Medical Letter*, said in 1971 that "vitamin E is of no value for *any* human ailment," and that has remained the point of view of many doctors ever since. As one skeptic commented, "Vitamin E is a vitamin in search of a disease."

There is no doubt that some of vitamin E's enthusiasts have often overstated the nutrient's value. Certainly, it will not make old men young, nor will it make impotent men sexy. But it does have its uses.

For example, a year after *Medical Letter* made its sweeping statement about the vitamin's inability to cure or curb any human afflictions, the National Research Council conceded that premature babies and people who have trouble absorbing fats require extra amounts of vitamin E. The following year several medical papers pointed out that vitamin E could improve circulation in the legs. Other reports by competent researchers have shown other uses for this long-little-known vitamin.

Two California physicians, Samuel Ayres, Jr., and Richard Mihan, both professors of medicine, have told of finding vitamin E useful in relieving nocturnal leg and foot cramps, as well as several other kinds of muscle spasm. They also report substantial success in treating several stubborn kinds of skin conditions with vitamin E. Some of their results have been confirmed by others. For example, a prominent Swedish surgeon, Dr. Kurt Haeger, says he has been able to reduce the number of leg amputations due to circulatory problems by 90 percent through giving his patients vitamin E.

In September 1972 the *American Journal of Clinical Nutrition* carried an article by two scientists and a physician indicating vitamin E's effectiveness in treating ulcers. The medical trio had been able to *greatly* reduce the range and intensity of induced ulcers in rats by giving them vitamin E before subjecting them to severe stress.

One interesting two-year study was conducted by a veterinarian in association with the manager of two Canadian stud farms. As told by Herbert Bailey in his book *Your Key to A Healthy Heart,* Dr. J. B. Chassels teamed up with F. G. Darlington, manager of the Windfields Farm and the National Stud Farm, both in Ontario, to see if vitamin E would improve the performance of the farms' racehorses. In two years, the farms' income went from $88,000 to over $196,000. The number of winners increased from eighty to ninety-five, while the number of second-place showings shot up from twenty-five to forty.

The most controversial claims made for vitamin E, however, center on its possibilities in helping heart problems. Two Canadian cardiologists, Doctors Wildred and Evan Shute, have been treating heart patients with vitamine E for several decades, and, they claim, with almost uniformly good results. Some American cardiologists, including the well-known and highly respected New Orleans specialist Dr. Alton Ochsner, have also found vitamin E useful in this respect. In a letter to the *New England Journal of Medicine* in 1964, Dr. Ochsner revealed, "In all patients in whom venous thrombosis might develop, for a number of years we have routinely prescribed Alpha Tocopherol [vitamin E]. . . ."

To be sure, some American researchers have pointed to experiments that tend to discredit such claims. In a study done at Cornell Medical College, nineteen heart patients received three hundred units of vitamin E a day for four months, while another nineteen received disguised placebos. The researchers reported no significant differences between the two groups. However, supporters of vitamin E maintain that the amount used in these and other such studies was too small. They point out that the Doctors Shute use dosages as high as 1,600 units or more a day. Dr. James P. Isaacs of Baltimore's Johns Hopkins University Hospital says that he has kept twenty-three out of twenty-five severely damaged heart patients alive for more than ten years with the use of vitamin E, vitamin C, and some mineral and hormonal supplements.

By this time, you may be wondering what all this had to do with vitamin E's possibilities as a protector against cancer. However, as we shall now see, some of the same properties that make the vitamin useful for these other ailments may also make it useful in our efforts to ward off malignant tissue.

To gain a better grasp of these properties, let us begin by considering what happens to an apple that has been cut in two. Right away the exposed pulp will start to turn brown. Why does it? Because it has come in contact with oxygen in the air. The same thing occurs with iron when it rusts or brass when it corrodes. Nearly all substances, including the human body, tend to fall prey sooner or later to the oxidation process.

Our atmosphere today abounds in oxidants. They include the ozone, the nitrogen oxide, and the halogens that are found in our air, especially when it is heavily polluted. They include the chlorine that is often added to our drinking water and the chlorine dioxide that is used to bleach flour for white bread. All of these substances may tend to make us "rust" a bit more, or a bit faster, than we might otherwise.

Fortunately, some substances also exist that tend to offset and oppose the oxidation process. They include two chemicals known as BHT and BHA, which are often used to preserve food from rotting. They include the mineral selenium as well as vitamin C and vitamin E. Of the two vitamins, vitamin E may be the most effective in this respect.

Vitamin E's ability to act as an antioxidant has been subjected to numerous tests. For example, at least three experiments have been done to see if the vitamin could protect laboratory animals from pollutants in the air. In all three experiments, vitamin E gave a good accounting of itself. In one of these experiments, which was reported in the March 1972 issue of *Journal of Agricultural and Food Chemistry,* the researchers found that rats given extra vitamin E would withstand the effects of various pollutants 50 to 100 percent longer than would rats that were deficient in the vitamin.

In recent years some scientists and physicians have started to wonder whether or not antioxidants, such as vitamin E, might prove to be protective against cancer. The reasoning behind such speculation is quite complex and need not concern us here. (It is based, upon other things, on the fact that oxidation products tend to increase at a cancer site, which in turn indicates that oxidation may play an important role in the formation of cancer.) At least two experiments that strengthen and support this speculation considerably have been reported.

The first of these experiments was carried out by Doctors Homer S. Black and Wan-Bang Lo at the Baylor College of Medicine in Houston. The two researchers wanted to see if antioxidants could prevent, or at least retard, the formation of a known cancer-causing substance that tends to build up on skin that has been heavily exposed to sunlight. They thus gave one group of mice a regular diet; another group a diet bolstered with antioxidants, including vitamin E. Subsequently, they irradiated the mice's skin to duplicate the effect of intense exposure to sunlight. Sure enough, the skin of the animals that had received the antioxidants contained, after two weeks, no detectable amounts of the carcinogen at all. The skin of the other mice showed evidence of its presence. (The carcinogen that they were looking for is called cholesterol alpha-oxide.)

This experiment was reported in a December 1973 issue

of *Nature*. Earlier that year, a group of researchers at the Cleveland Clinic Foundation reported the results of another, and potentially more significant, experiment in the *Proceedings of the National Academy of Sciences*. The researchers took as the basis of their investigation the widely held belief that cancer begins with damage to the chromosome of the cell. They wanted to see if antioxidants could protect cells from the damage wrought by cancer-causing agents.

They administered a carcinogen called OMBA to some human blood cells taken from a volunteer donor. As predicted, the cells experienced substantial chromosomal breaks. However, they found that when they added the antioxidant chemical, BHT, to the carcinogen, they reduced such breakage by more than two-thirds. They then tried adding vitamin C to the carcinogen. This reduced the damage by 31.7 percent, not nearly as much as was achieved through BHT, but a substantial drop nonetheless. The mineral selenium proved to be still more effective than vitamin C, as it reduced the damage by 41 percent. Most effective of all the natural and nutritional anti-oxidants used in the experiment was vitamin E. It scored a 63.2 percent decrease in cellular damage.

Commenting on the results of their experiment, the scientists expressed the belief that "the protection against chromosomal breakage provided by antioxidants may have important relationships to aging and carcinogenesis [cancer formation]." Indeed, it *could* signal a vital breakthrough in cancer prevention and even treatment, and it points up the possibilities of vitamin E.

You will note that the scientists, in their concluding comment on their experiment, pointed to its potential value, not only in terms of cancer, but also in terms of aging. Cancer and aging are obviously correlated, for as one ages, one becomes more vulnerable to malignancy. However, they may also be more directly related. Whatever keeps the cells

of the body more youthful is likely to keep them less susceptible to cancer.

In this connection we should note that antioxidants have
also demonstrated a capacity to prolong the life span. Dr.
Denham Harman, a professor of medicine at the University
of Nebraska College of Medicine, has increased the life span
of laboratory animals by nearly 50 percent by giving them
the antioxidant chemicals BHT and BHA. Vitamin E has also
shown some ability to lengthen life. Giving extra vitamin E to
animals has increased, at least slightly, their longevity. Dr.
Ayres, the California medical school professor whose use of
vitamin E to alleviate a variety of ailments was cited earlier,
points to another possible aspect of the relationship between
vitamin E and aging. He has observed that the chemistry of a
rare disease called progeria, in which a child may age twenty
years for each year of his or her life, suggests that this
strange malady may stem from an inability to utilize vitamin E.

One more experiment in regard to vitamin E's capacity
to maintain cellular health is also worthy of note. Two scientists from the Lawrence Berkeley Laboratory of the University of California cultured two groups of cells from a human
lung. They added vitamin E to one of the groups but not to
the other. The cells in the group that did not receive the
vitamin reproduced themselves 50 times and then died. The
cells receiving the vitamin E, however, were still thriving
after having reproduced themselves 120 times!

In an interview with medical writer Harold J. Taub of
Prevention magazine, the scientists took great pains to point
out that what happens in a laboratory does not necessarily
happen in the functioning human body, and that, therefore,
their experiment did not necessarily mean that vitamin E
would make people live longer. However, when Taub ques-
tioned them further, he found that ever since the experiment, each of them has been taking 200 units of vitamin E a
day.

Summary

We have in this chapter covered a lot of ground in a brief and, perhaps, somewhat bewildering manner. Nevertheless, the essential lessons to be drawn from the material presented should be reasonably clear. Vitamins A, B, and E belong in everyone's anticancer arsenal. While the evidence on vitamin A is, so far, somewhat more sizable and specific than the evidence on vitamin E, both show unmistakable signs of being able to help the human body stave off malignancy. And while disagreement exists as to which of the B vitamins may have the greatest role to play in counteracting cancer, we can avoid the problems, and other possible problems as well, by simply taking them all.

In Chapter 9, entitled "Living the Anticancer Life," we will look at such questions as desirable amounts of dosages and natural versus synthetic vitamins, along with the foods that best supply them. It is now time to turn to another set of substances that can help us hold malignancy at bay.

5

Minerals That Help You Resist Cancer

Most people are much less aware of minerals than they are of vitamins. When they do think of minerals, they usually confine their attention to calcium and iron. But minerals play an important role in human nutrition. Furthermore, there are many more minerals that are vital to human health than calcium and iron. And it is some of the less well-known minerals that help protect us from cancer.

Magnesium: The Mighty Mineral

Early in this century a French physician named Pierre Delbert began to have doubts about the antiseptics that he and his colleagues were using to heal wounds. These antiseptics might help kill the infection, but, he speculated, they also might damage the cells that fight infection.

As an army surgeon during World War I, Dr. Delbert found his fears tragically confirmed. Medicine had now identified the white blood cells as the body's own infection fighters, and, sure enough, the antiseptics seemed to damage them severely. This finding prompted Delbert to launch an intensive search for something that would strengthen these cells. He finally found it, he felt, in a compound called magnesium chloride.

Dr. Delbert began giving injections of magnesium chloride solution to the wounded soldiers under his care. The results proved reassuring to both him and his nurses. After some time, he began wondering if the compound could not be administered orally. His nurses smilingly told him that they were certain that it could be, because they had begun drinking it themselves. They had noticed how the magnesium chloride seemed to strengthen the patients, and being overworked and in need of some extra strength, they had started to imbibe it with uniformly good effects.

Delbert not only began giving it to his patients orally, but taking a tip from his nurses, started to drink it himself. He was pleased with the results. After the war, he refined and improved his new medicine by adding to it other magnesium compounds. He used it in treating a variety of ailments, including diphtheria, typhoid, and infantile paralysis. He also continued to take it regularly himself.

Here, one of the many ironies of modern medicine reveals itself. Although Delbert went on to win prominence and prestige—he became a hospital department head, a professor of medicine, and the author of several standard French medical texts—his work with magnesium never evoked much enthusiasm. Indeed, many French doctors showed little awareness of it. When he died in 1957, at the age of ninety-six, his lengthy obituaries listed many of his accomplishments but scarcely mentioned magnesium chloride.

Fortunately, a few doctors, both in France and elsewhere, had become interested in the workings of this little-known and little-appreciated mineral. A year after Dr. Delbert's death, the highly respected Canadian physician Hans Selye of McGill University published research showing that magnesium could greatly aid rats in surviving severe stress brought on by subjecting them to extreme cold. In Dr. Selye's experiment, all the rats not given magnesium died from the cold, while all the rats receiving the magnesium survived. In analyzing this and other experiments he conducted along the same line, Selye came to the conclusion that magnesium checks the development of cholesterol, though it actually becomes used up in the process.

On the heels of his investigatory work, much more research began coming to light on the beneficial effects of magnesium on matters relating to the heart. One study showed that people dying from a heart attack had much less magnesium in their hearts than did those who died from other causes. Also, the more severe the attack, the less magnesium the organ contained. Another study showed that people living in communities with hard water, which contains a good deal of magnesium as well as calcium, suffered substantially fewer heart attacks than those living in communities where the drinking water was soft. Nebraska, for example, has more hard water than any other state, and its death rate from heart attacks is one-third the national average. (In England it was found that those communities that switched from hard water to soft soon began experiencing a rise in heart disease.) High blood pressure also seemed to be helped by magnesium.

One interesting example of the role of magnesium in human health, and of the tendency of modern medicine to overlook this role, comes from Finland. One of Finland's northeastern provinces gained fame in the 1960s as the land of the beautiful widows. It seems that the province's menfolk, despite the fact that most of them led a vigorous outdoor life—their principal occupation was lumberjacking—were experiencing the highest rate of heart attacks in the world. Their rate of death from heart attack was three times that of men in the United States.

The United Nations World Health Organization got together with the Finnish government to initiate a five-year study project to see what caused this phenomenon. They soon felt they had the answer. The men were eating too much saturated fat, smoking too many cigarettes, and drinking too much beer. However, the researchers forgot something. The health habits of the province's men may not have been the best, but they were not all that different from those of other Finnish men or, for that matter, American men. On February 1, 1974, *Medical World News* carried what may prove to be the answer. The province's soil, so two Finnish investigators had found, contains only about one-third as much available magnesium as the soil in the southwestern part of the country.

If modern-day medicine tends to neglect the role of magnesium in helping the heart, it has shown itself even less cognizant of the role magnesium can play in cancer prevention. The evidence of the part magnesium can play in this regard may not be quite complete, but is nevertheless quite compelling.

The long road connecting magnesium to cancer begins in France. However, though Dr. Delbert thought that his prized magnesium remedy might act as a "brake on cancer," it fell to another French physician to point to the first possible linkage. Since the beginning of the century there had been reports that Egypt had an extremely low cancer rate, and a Parisian doctor named P. Schrumpf-Pierron decided to see if, and why, this was true.

He found that Egyptians had a cancer rate only one-tenth that of Europeans, even though Europeans were better nourished. Furthermore, when cancer did develop in an Egyptian, it was likely to develop less quickly and to display less of a tendency to spread. Investigating further, Schrumpf-Pierron found that thanks to soil conditions and possibly other factors, the average Egyptian consumed about five or six times as much magnesium as the average European.

The French physician then decided to test his theory in his own country. Sure enough he found that in those parts of France where the soil was comparatively rich in magnesium, the cancer rate tended to be low. Where the soil was poor in magnesium, the cancer rate tended to be high.

We might want to question some of the doctor's findings. For example, he claimed that potassium was the real cancer culprit and that magnesium's value lay in its ability to counteract potassium. This, of course, runs contrary to Dr. Gerson's theory and experience, as we saw in chapter 2. But his principal postulate, that magnesium deficiency may lead to cancerous growth, has found some distinguished and rather decisive support in recent years.

In 1968 Dr. P. Bois, an M.D. and Ph.D. from the University of Montreal, revealed that he had induced tumors in rats by simply feeding them a magnesium-free diet for two months. As he put it in a talk to the Federation of American Societies for Experimental Biology, "Withdrawing magnesium may lead to mutation of chromosomes and the mutation may lead to tumors."

His work confirmed what four Chicago physicians had reported earlier in the *Journal of the American Medical Association.* They found, in working with rats, that giving the animals a *marginally* magnesium-deficient diet produced leukemia (cancer of the blood) in 10 percent of them after about eight months. What makes this experiment more interesting is that they had chosen a species of rat that had generally shown itself resistant to leukemia. The leukemia that the rats developed was indistinguishable from the leukemia that affects human beings.

The physicians continued to experiment by giving chemicals known to produce leukemia and/or other forms of cancer to rats that had been fed with varying amounts of magnesium. Those rats that had received magnesium-rich diets actually seemed to be immune from leukemia, although some of them did develop other forms of cancer. The leader of the research team, Dr. George M. Hass, chairman of the pathology department of Rush-Presbyterian-St. Luke's Medical Center, subsequently told *Prevention* magazine, "It has become apparent to us that the magnesium-deficient animals have a greatly reduced ability to destroy the tumor cells."

More recent research points to some of the reasons that magnesium tends to act as a cancer controller. A 1975 Iowa State University study showed that rats fed a magnesium-deficient diet produced fewer antibodies, while other studies have indicated that lack of magnesium curtails the action of lymphocytes, which constitute another of the body's defense systems against foreign invaders. Dr. Alan D. Mease of the Walter Reed Army Medical Center says this weakening of the lymphocyte-cellular immunization system may be the reason that magnesium-deficient rats seem so prone to certain malignancies.

For Dr. Harry Rubin, Professor of Molecular Biology at the University of California at Berkeley, the role of magnesium is crucial to the proper functioning of the living cell. He has found that when the cell's supply of magnesium becomes drastically reduced, its metabolic functions start to limp and lag. "Magnesium," he said in an interview published in the July 1976 issue of *Prevention*, "is the only substance that has an effect on every pathway to the cell." It is, he said, the "universal controller" to all cell life. And let us not forget that cancer is primarily a cellular disturbance.

Important as magnesium seems to be in curbing cancer, we should not overestimate its value. As we shall see in a later chapter, the nutritionist Adelle Davis took plenty of magnesium and still died of cancer. Nevertheless, the available research does indicate that magnesium can help us in triumphing over this disease. Indications are that those who let themselves become deficient in this mineral lay themselves especially open to the development of malignant tumor growth.

This last point looms in importance when we examine the typical American diet. It supplies around 300 to 350 milligrams of magnesium a day. However, the Food and Nutrition Board has established a recommended daily allowance for adult males at 400 milligrams a day, while Dr. Mildred S. Seelig, who has done extensive research in this area, feels the figure should be higher. Dr. Seelig claims that the average man needs 500 milligrams a day and teenagers and pregnant women may require more. According to Dr. Seelig, the average American needs at least 200 more milligrams of magnesium every day than he customarily gets to keep himself or herself in the best of health. Dr. Roger J. Williams has expressed a similar concern, "It seems clear that [with most Americans] magnesium deficiency is not only a possibility but a probability."

The fact is that magnesium is an easily available, but also an easily destroyable, mineral. There is, for example, plenty of magnesium in wheat, but most of it gets discarded when we process the wheat into bleached white flour. A slice of white bread has actually lost about 85 percent of its magnesium. Similarly, white rice has less than one-third the magnesium of brown rice and frosted peas have one-third less magnesium than raw peas. Breast milk is quite rich in magnesium; cow's milk has much less; and pasteurized cow's milk has very little. Thus, most American babies begin life with a less-than-desirable amount of this vital mineral.

Furthermore, many things that we do eat cause us to lose

magnesium. Meat, alcohol, and sugar, for instance, all tend
to use up magnesium in the body. Even milk can reduce the
availability of magnesium. Generally, the more calcium one
consumes, the more magnesium one should have, and vice
versa, since the two minerals seem to be interdependent.
Milk drinkers who do not maintain a high intake of magnesium may become especially prone to magnesium deficiency.

Fortunately, there are still many foods, as well as food
supplements, that provide magnesium in generous amounts.
They include wheat germ and whole wheat products generally, buckwheat and cottonseed flour, red hot chili peppers,
egg yolks, blackstrap molasses, bananas, some beans, and
most nuts and seeds. Supplements from health food stores
are available in the form of dolomite, which provides calcium
along with the magnesium, magnesium oxide tablets and
powder, and in other forms as well. The concerned cancer-
preventer will make sure that his or her system is kept well
supplied with this mighty mineral.

Selenium: The "Sleeper" Mineral

Twenty-odd years ago, if you asked a nutrition-oriented
chemist or physician about selenium, you would have received a blank look accompanied by a shrug of the shoulders.
Few medical workers at that time had even heard of the
mineral. However, if you happened to stumble upon one
who had, the chances are that the response to your inquiry
would have produced a horrified look and a stern warning to
keep away from selenium. In one sense, such a response
would have been justified. Selenium, in substantial amounts,
can be quite injurious to any living thing.

But there is another side to selenium, and it is one that has been receiving increasing attention in recent years. Science has shown that many substances can both kill *and* cure—that what may be most damaging in large doses can be most desirable in smaller ones. It appears that such is the case with selenium.

As far back as 1915 there was speculation that selenium might be an anticancer agent. In 1949 some research was reported showing that rats receiving selenium supplementation developed tumors more slowly once they were exposed to a cancer-producing chemical. However, like so many early studies showing a relationship between dietary supplementation and cancer control, this one went largely ignored.

Selenium only started to really attract attention in the late 1950s when Dr. Klaus Schwarz, a physician at the University of California School of Medicine, found that it could preserve the liver tissue of laboratory rats from fatal destruction. When Dr. Schwarz first isolated the protecting substance he thought he had stumbled across a new vitamin. Only upon closer examination did he and his co-workers find that the protector was the little-known mineral selenium.

Subsequent research showed that selenium could protect animals from other situations and substances that could do them grave injury. The best known of these came to light during the great fish scare of 1970. In that year the U.S. government halted the sale of swordfish and canned tuna fish after finding levels of mercury in the fish that were considered to be toxic. The ban was lifted, however, when research revealed that the fish had always contained such theoretically high levels of mercury, but that the selenium present in the fish had rendered this mercury harmless to human beings.

Selenium came into its own as an anticancer agent in 1973 when Dr. Raymond Shamberger reported the rather startling results of a survey of thirty-four roughly similar

American cities. He found that in the seventeen cities located in comparatively high selenium areas, the cancer death rate amounted to 127 per 100,000 population. But the cancer death rate in those cities with less selenium came to 175. The *lowest* cancer death rate occurred in the city with the *highest* selenium soil content, Rapid City, South Dakota.

In June 1973 the same month that Dr. Shamberger revealed the results of his selenium survey in the *Medical Tribune*, the *Journal of Nutrition* published an article summarizing the results of some laboratory experiments with selenium. The laboratory findings dovetailed with Shamberger's city survey, for they showed that supplying selenium to test animals markedly increased their resistance to cancer.

Rounding out the record came further research showing an even more direct link between selenium and cancer in human beings. A test of one thousand patients showed that those with the highest incidence of cancer had the lowest levels of selenium in their blood. Commenting on this Dr. John L. Martin of Colorado State University told *Prevention*, "The results were startling. There was a positive inverse relationship between cancer involvement and serum selenium."

Selenium's ability to combat cancer may be attributed in part to the fact that it is an antioxidant. As we saw in the previous chapter, the Cleveland Clinic Foundation study of antioxidants and cancer control tested selenium with favorable results. However, the mineral may possess other anti-cancer properties as well. Dr. Martin has found, to his amazement, that mice fed selenium produce twenty to thirty times as many antibodies as mice fed a normal diet. As another scientist has observed, selenium is "a real ham," for everything it does is dramatic.

If you live in Texas or New Mexico, you are likely to be consuming more selenium than if you live in New York State or Pennsylvania. But wherever you live, if you are concerned with cancer prevention, you will want to make sure you get enough selenium in your diet.

Two of the richest selenium sources are sesame seeds and wheat germ. Another good source is brewer's yeast. Eggs also contain some useful amounts of this important mineral. Seafood generally supplies more selenium than meat, with shrimp, lobster, smelts, and tuna heading the list. Two kinds of meat, kidneys and liver, offer sizable amounts of selenium. (Kidneys contain four times as much selenium as liver, but liver contains four times as much as other kinds of meat.)

Vegetables are generally poor sources of selenium, but there are exceptions. Garlic and mushrooms are reasonably rich in selenium, while asparagus also has appreciable quantities of the mineral.

As noted at the outset, too much selenium can be dangerous. Those who have studied it, however, feel that this should not worry anyone who obtains his selenium supply from natural sources. Dr. Schwarz, who has been researching the mineral since the 1950s, feels that the average American could double his current consumption of selenium without endangering his health. It seems likely that such an increased intake could pay off with an increased degree of health and a decreased rate of cancer.

Iodine

It is well known that breast cancer is the leading cause of cancer death among women. What causes this particular form of cancer, however, is not well known. Dr. Bernhard A. Eskin, chief of the Gynecologic Endocrinology Service at the Albert Einstein Medical Center in Philadelphia, feels he has an answer to at least part of the problem. And what he has to say is well worth listening to.

Dr. Eskin believes that a definite and distinct relationship exists between breast cancer and a deficiency of iodine. His brief is based on both laboratory research and statistical data. In his laboratory he has injected substantial amounts of the potent carcinogen DMBA into rats kept on iodine-deficient diets. Almost invariably they developed malignant breast tumors substantially sooner than did rats that had received an adequate supply of iodine in their diets.

A statistical survey he has made further backs up his belief. He has noticed that the highest death rate from breast cancer in this country occurs in the Great Lakes region. This region is also known as the Goiter Belt because of its lack of iodine. The same statistical correlations also show up in a country-by-country survey. Breast cancer, he points out, tends to be most prevalent in those nations that tend to be iodine-deficient. In countries like Japan, however, where iodine consumption tends to be relatively high, breast cancer tends to be relatively low.

Can iodine actually be used in treating breast cancer? Dr. Eskin does not say so, but he does report treating ten women who suffered from what is called breast dysplasia. Breast dysplasia results from abnormal changes in the breast tissue that produce nodules, cysts, and benign tumors. About one in every four American women suffer from breast dysplasia at some time during their life, and while a majority of them never contract breast cancer, they become, statistically, four times as likely to do so as other women. Breast dysplasia is thus considered a precancerous condition.

Dr. Eskin reports that his ten breast dysplasia patients all responded positively to iodine therapy. After adequate iodine intake, their dysplasia decreased and, in some instances, disappeared altogether. "The treatment," Eskin told the National Medical Association at its 1971 convention, "seemed to be effective and at least temporarily improved the breast condition."

We should be careful not to read too much into his findings. He is certainly not suggesting that he has a cure for breast cancer. What he is suggesting is that anyone who fails to maintain an adequate intake of iodine is running a much greater risk of coming down with this malignancy.

Men as well as women could do well to heed the lessons of Eskin's research. For one thing, breast cancer can occur in men, though it rarely happens. More importantly, however, any internal condition that may tend to produce cancer at one site in the body possesses at least the possibility of producing the same condition at another site. Dr. Gerson, it will be recalled, made sure all his patients received an adequate iodine intake by making Lugol's solution a part of their diets.

Iodine is not the most readily available mineral, but it is found in most seafood. (Fresh water fish has much less.) It can also be obtained from kelp tablets, which are available in health food stores. Another, but less satisfactory, source is iodized salt. The trouble here is that one usually has to use too much salt to obtain the necessary amount of iodine, and since Americans are already oversalted, so to speak, it is best to seek out other sources. Iodine, except possibly in exorbitant amounts, is not toxic, and Dr. Eskin's research, as well as Dr. Gerson's record, indicates that it is better to consume too much rather than too little of this apparently anticancer agent.

Zinc

In its December 1969 issue, the *National Hog Farmer* reported that many of the nation's pigs were starting to show symptoms of severe stress. Some were even going into convulsions and dying. The reason? Less and less zinc in their feed. Two scientists, Doctors Robert F. Keefer and Rabindar N. Singh, revealed that sweet corn grown in soil heavily fertilized with artificial fertilizers had been found especially susceptible to a loss of this trace mineral. The decreased amount of zinc in the corn given to the pigs was primarily responsible for their stress symptoms.

It is rather tragically typical that the first alarm to be sounded on the loss of an important mineral in food resulted from concern about how the loss was affecting animals, not human beings. As a nation, we tend to show much more concern over animal nutrition than human nutrition. Such was the case when the lowering of zinc levels in crops was first noticed.

Zinc is not only important for pigs but also for man. Deficiencies in this trace element can stunt the growth of sex organs and even of the whole body. Indeed, certain types of dwarfs grow to normal size when given extra amounts of zinc. Lack of zinc can also slow down the healing of wounds, reduce the sense of smell, and contribute to prostate and ulcer conditions. Zinc even seems to have an effect on the human personality, for a deficiency in the mineral can cause lethargy and listlessness. One psychiatrist, Dr. Carl C. Pfeiffer of the New Jersey Neuro-psychiatric Institute, says that inadequate zinc could be a factor in at least some cases of schizophrenia.

Zinc may also have something to do with intelligence. Tests consistently show that people with higher levels of zinc in their bodies also tend to have higher I.Q.'s than those with lower levels of the mineral.

At least two respected researchers have expressed considerable concern over a decline of zinc in the American diet. One of these was Henry Schroeder, M.D., who for many years headed the trace mineral laboratory at Dartmouth Medical College. As director of the only laboratory concentrating on trace minerals, Dr. Schroeder was an expert on the role of zinc in human nutrition. The other specialist is Donald Oberlas, Ph.D., a biochemist at Wayne State University School of Medicine in Detroit.

Working independently of each other, both men came to the conclusion that zinc deficiency was becoming a serious problem. The deficiency may be caused not only by the use of artificial fertilizer, but by the processing of food. Wheat, for example, loses 78 percent of its zinc when converted into bleached white flour. Alcohol and even sugar may deplete zinc from the body.

Just as a zinc deficiency can make certain medical problems worse, zinc supplementation can sometimes make them better. An increased intake of zinc can help alleviate prostate and ulcer symptoms, sharpen sense of smell, and cause wounds to heal more rapidly.

This last-named feature of zinc indicates a possible use in controlling cancer. A small, but quite suggestive, body of evidence now exists to support such speculation. The *Lancet* of June 9, 1973, carried a communication from H. Kirchner of the National Cancer Institute pointing out that zinc supplements tend to stimulate the supply of infection-fighting lymphocytes in the blood. What's more, the mineral was able to accomplish this without any observable side effects.

Another respected British journal, *Nature,* had previously carried in its June 18, 1971, issue a report more specifically linking zinc to cancer control. In an experiment, rats given zinc supplements showed added ability to withstand the effects of a cancer-causing agent. Zinc, concluded the writer, "seems to exert an inhibitory effect on tumor formation."

If you wish to increase your intake of zinc, then your best bet for doing so is to eat more herring and oysters. Both are remarkably rich in this mineral. Oysters found along the Atlantic coast contain more than twice as much zinc as those found along the Pacific shore, but even oysters from the Pacific supply goodly amounts of the mineral. Herring is a much cheaper source and is more available than you might think, since most American sardines are really small herrings. Most seafood, especially shellfish, offers appreciable amounts of zinc, as do eggs, wheat germ, and most meats. Zinc supplements are available in most health food stores and in some drugstores.

Molybdenum

Molybdenum, another trace element, also seems to have some relationship with cancer. This is the opinion of Dr. John Berg of the National Cancer Institute. In his remarks to the Seventh National Cancer Institute in 1972, Dr. Berg noted that in a region of South Africa called Transkei, where cancer of the esophagus has shot upwards in recent years, researchers have found great deficiencies of molybdenum in the region's plants. Meanwhile, surveys in this country show a high incidence of cancer of the esophagus in areas where the water supply is deficient in molybdenum.

Molybdenum is found most abundantly in legumes such as peas and various kinds of beans, whole-grain cereals, leafy vegetables, and our old friends, liver and kidney. As in the case of so many other valuable nutrients, refining and processing tends to rob foods of their molybdenum content. White flour, for example, contains only half the amount of this mineral as whole wheat.

Other trace minerals may also be of use in curbing cancer. Dr. Erwin Dilyan, in his book *Vitamins in Your Life*, says platinum compounds have inhibited certain cancers in mice. More importantly, in his view, platinum, as well as palladium, increases the effectiveness of anticancer drugs. However, Dilyan fails to mention any natural sources for these trace minerals, so most of us will have to forego any benefits they might bestow.

Chromium

Another trace mineral that has begun to arouse increased interest in the nutritional community in recent years is chromium. Most of the research regarding it has been done by the Trace Mineral Laboratory at Dartmouth Medical School. And what researchers there have found out about it warrants the attention of any health-oriented person.

Apparently, only the most minute quantities of chromium are needed by the human body. But if the body does not receive, and retain, this tiny amount, it may well develop problems. These problems are generally of an arteriosclerotic nature. However, chromium also appears to play a role in aging. For example, a group of rats fed a chromium-enriched diet lived for four years. In the words of the laboratory's director, Dr. Henry Schroeder, this probably set a new record in rat longevity. Since longevity, as we have seen, often relates to reduced risk of cancer, we should take care to see that we obtain enough chromium.

The problem with chromium is that many of the foods and beverages that have become such mainstays of the modern American diet tend to strip chromium from the body. What are these chromium-depriving foods? Alcohol, sugar, and white flour are the principal ones. Consumed over long periods of time they tend to decrease the already microscopic amounts of chromium that we have.

What foods tend to enrich the body's supply of this trace

mineral? One of the best is brewer's yeast, a food that, as we have seen and shall continue to see, contains so many other nourishing nutrients. Fruit juices, especially grape juice, also contain ample amounts of chromium. From this we may infer that the fruits themselves, especially grapes and raisins, will similarly build up our body's chromium reserves. And although white sugar makes us lose chromium, honey and molasses have the opposite effect. Dr. Schroeder found that even brown sugar, which is simply sugar covered with molasses, could increase rather than decrease the amount of chromium in the body, providing the sugar was so brown that it would tend to stick together and be hard to pour.

Since the chromium problem confronts us with an increasingly familiar list of nutritional friends and foes, it should pose no great difficulties. Eating foods rich in chromium, and eschewing foods that tend to be chromium-depleting, will not only increase our stores of chromium itself but provide us with various other valuable nutrients as well.

Sulfur

A former co-worker once told me about her grandfather who had remained vigorous and active up to his death at the age of ninety-seven. My first reaction, naturally enough, was to ask her what he ate. His two favorite foods, she replied, were horseradish and red hot peppers. This reminded me of another horseradish buff, Konrad Adenauer. Adenauer served as prime minister of West Germany until he was in his late eighties. Even in his nineties he was still generating enough work to keep two secretaries fully occupied.

Interestingly and intriguing though they may be, two cases of men eating horseradish and staying active into their nineties does not constitute valid evidence of anything in particular, and so I let the matter rest. However, in the spring of 1976 Dr. Carl C. Pfeiffer published a book entitled *Mental and Elemental Nutrients, A Physician's Guide to Nutrition and Health Care* that made me think again. Dr. Pfeiffer, you may recall, is the nutrition-oriented psychiatrist who was quoted as suspecting that certain types of schizophrenics suffer from a zinc deficiency. In his book, Dr. Pfeiffer talks about a lot of things besides zinc. One of them is sulfur.

Sulfur, according to Dr. Pfeiffer, is not a trace mineral, since an adult, so he claims, needs about 850 milligrams daily to stay healthy. Every cell of our body contains sulfur and needs continual replenishment of the mineral to function with optimum effectivemess. Although no scientific study has yet been reported linking sulfur deficiency to cancer, anything that preserves and protects the body's cells can assist it in fighting cancer. Furthermore, sulfur seems to have some relationship to selenium, whose anticancer properties we have already examined.

Where do we find sulfur? You have probably already guessed part of the answer. Horseradish and red hot peppers are two excellent sources, as are garlic, onions, and eggs. What about sulfur supplements? They are available but they are designated and designed only for cattle, pigs, and chickens. This is yet another tragic reminder that we have been more concerned with keeping animals healthy than we have human beings.

Potassium

Lastly, we come to the mineral on which Dr. Gerson based so much of his diet. As it happens, no scientific evidence has ever emerged indicating that potassium can protect the human body from cancer. It may well be that the effectiveness of Gerson's diet stemmed from the other nutrients that it contained. We will never know until proper tests of potassium's behavior in the face of cancer have been made.

Potassium, in any case, does have a contribution to make to human health, for it aids the functioning of the heart and muscles. Since overall health is important in any anticancer regimen, and since Dr. Gerson may someday be proved right in giving it a prominent position in the body's fight against cancer, we should all make sure that we get enough potassium.

That many of us may not be obtaining sufficient supplies of this mineral has been suggested by two different, and quite distinguished, sources. The *Journal of the American Medical Association* published a report in its October 6, 1969, issue pointing out that muscle weakness was usually one of the first symptoms of potassium deficiency. The two physicians who authored the report expressed the belief that older people are especially likely to lack this mineral. Earlier that year, as if to confirm this fear, *Geriatric Focus* published the results of a careful survey of senior citizens taken near Glasgow, Scotland. The survey found that 52 percent of these elderly people were not getting all the potassium they needed.

While older persons may be especially prone to potassium deficiencies, younger people are by no means immune. The three astronauts who went to the moon were all found, on their return, to be deficient in the mineral—thanks, in part, to their having been given a commercial vitamin C drink instead of real orange juice. Keep in mind that potassium is somewhat perishable, in that alcohol, salt, stress of various kinds, and certain drugs all tend to flush potassium out of our bodies.

Potassium is not hard to obtain. It is especially plentiful in fruit. Bananas and oranges are two prime sources; apples and grapes are also good.

6

Foods for the Fight

Food constitutes, perhaps, our primary weapon against cancer. What we eat and, as we shall see in a later chapter, what we don't eat may well make the difference in how well we can meet the menace of cancer, this now-sweeping scourge. Those foods that help us develop our defenses against cancer do so largely because of the vitamins and minerals they contain. But some foods seem to possess additional properties that act to curb and control the growth of malignant tumors.

Liver

Over twenty-five years ago, in July 1951, a medical publication entitled *Proceedings of the Society of Experimental Biology and Medicine* carried the report of an intriguing, indeed exciting, experiment carried out by a scientist named Benjamin H. Ershoff. Dr. Ershoff, so it seems, had started to wonder if liver did not house some special ingredient, beyond the numerous B vitamins that it contains, that might fight fatigue. In an effort to find out, he took three different groups of rats and fed them three different diets over a period of twelve weeks. The first group received the basic laboratory diet plus some extra vitamins. The second group got the first group's diet with a generous supply of B vitamins added to it. The third group was given the first group's diet, but instead of the extra B vitamins, 10 percent of the diet was replaced by desiccated (dried) liver.

Dr. Ershoff then dropped all three groups into a tank of water where they had to keep swimming or drown. The results? The first two groups of rats lasted a little less than 13½ minutes before giving up. But the group that had received the heavy liver supplementation fared much much better. Of the twelve rats in this group, one swam for 13 minutes, one for 83 minutes, and one for 87 minutes. What about the other nine? They were still swimming at the end of two hours when Dr. Ershoff ended the experiment. He had found what he wanted to find out. There is something special about, or rather in, liver.

As it so happens, the same month the *Proceedings* reported Dr. Ershoff's experiment, the *Journal of Nutrition* carried the article by Dr. Kanematsu Sugiura reporting on his efforts to control cancer through dietary means. One food that he used with substantial success, as we saw when we examined the possibilities of B vitamins in cancer control, was brewer's yeast. Another food substance that Dr. Sugiura experimented with was desiccated liver. The liver actually proved more potent than the brewer's yeast in curbing cancer growth. With brewer's yeast, you may recall, it was necessary to replace 15 percent of the rats' normal diet for absolute protection. With liver, only a 10 percent ration was necessary to ensure that none of the rats that were fed the carcinogen developed liver cancer.

Subsequent research showed that liver in the diet could act as an antidote to some powerful poisons and pollutants such as strychnine, sulfanilamide, and some other noxious chemicals. In other words, liver contained some detoxifying component.

In July 1971 a team of biochemists at the University of Michigan Medical Center proudly announced that they had isolated and identified the special substance in liver that was responsible for all of its good works. They described this as a red protein pigment which they called Cytochrome P-450. In a press release on July 13, Dr. Minor J. Coon, who headed the team, said, "Cytochrome P-450 may prove to be part of the solution to pollution, drug addiction, alcoholism, and even cancer."

Some ten months later, another news item from Michigan added substance to such a claim. Dr. Albert Szent-Gyorgyi, the research physician who won the Nobel prize for discovering vitamin C, spoke before an audience at Wayne State University in Detroit. He reported finding that laboratory mice that were fed extracts of liver developed a remarkable resistance to cancer. He claimed to have spotlighted a special substance in liver that fulfilled this function. He called this compound "retine." Said the Nobel laureate, "We are on the verge of finding the key to curing cancer."

Unfortunately, however, the National Institutes of Health turned down his application for funds to continue his research. The Institutes was more interested in spending the many millions of government dollars that it had at its disposal on the search for anticancer drugs instead.

However, this does not prevent us from making liver part of our own defense network against cancer. Even if it does not contain any special ingredient, it remains a treasure chest of vitamins, minerals, and other substances that tend to inhibit cancer. A 3½-ounce portion of beef liver contains over 50,000 units of vitamin A and 250 micrograms of folic acid, a B vitamin that has often been linked to anticancer activity. (You may recall from our earlier discussion of B vitamins in chapter 4 that folic acid was the B vitamin most often cited as an anticancer agent.) Liver also contains at least a moderate amount of selenium and a substantial amount of nucleic acid, whose potential role in cancer protection we will examine later on. Dried liver in either tablet or powdered form contains all, or almost all, the anticancer benefits of regular liver in concentrated amounts. It is available at health food stores.

Fiber

Lung cancer is the number one cancer killer of men; breast cancer is the number one cancer killer of women. But the cancer that rates as the number two killer for both sexes is cancer of the bowel and colon. As a matter of fact, it runs a close second to lung cancer in the country's overall cancer mortality rate. Some 76,000 Americans die each year from this malignancy.

In January 1971 a well-known and well-respected British physician named Denis Burkitt offered a new theory regarding its causes to a group of cancer specialists meeting in San Diego. Dr. Burkitt, known for his discovery of Burkitt's lymphoma among other things, had spent some time studying the diet and diseases of native African people. He noted that they ate a diet that was high in roughage or fiber, that is, substances that are not absorbed into the body itself but are expelled through the waste system. As a result, the Africans that he had studied customarily moved their bowels twice a day, each time evacuating large, but almost odor-free, stools. Indeed, when one of these people failed to have two bowel movements during the day, he considered himself to be ill.

Dr. Burkitt also found something else characteristic of these people. They hardly ever suffered from colitis, diverticular disease, or cancer of the bowel or colon. The British physician, along with the other physicians who were assisting him in his study, concluded that the two different phenomena were strongly related. A high residue diet, one in which there is much leftover food to discharge through the bowels, tends to protect people from such cancer.

Dr. Burkitt also offered an opinion as to why this is so. Fecal matter, he said, may very well contain one or more cancer-causing substances. When a diet is low in roughage, as is that of Western man, this matter stays in the bowels longer. Furthermore, without the roughage to provide bulk, the cancer-causing substances become more concentrated.

Burkitt's findings triggered a great deal of research, most of which tended to substantiate his claims. For example, two other British physicians reported in the November 3, 1973, *British Medical Journal* that bran, a food very high in fiber, tends to prevent colonic bacteria from transforming bile salts into cancer-causing substances. Two years later the National Cancer Institute found that people suffering from cancer of the colon tend to consume considerably less fibrous foods than do those who remain free of this ailment.

Fortunately this is one cancer preventive that has succeeded in arousing some public attention and acceptance. This is in part due to a book written by a California psychiatrist named David Reuben. Dr. Reuben's interest became aroused when he had to go through the agony of watching his own father die of colonic cancer. He began to read up on the literature and wrote a best-seller called *The Save-Your-Life-Diet*. In this book he points out that a diet high in roughage not only can prevent cancer of the digestive tract, but can also deter other digestive problems including constipation. Furthermore, there is even research to suggest that fiber tends to lower cholesterol.

Of course, not all doctors are yet convinced. Speaking of bran, for example, the *Journal of the American Medical Association* said, in an editorial, "Until its health benefits become firmly established, its discomfort and lack of aesthetic appeal will preclude widespread use." This statement prompted nutritionist Dr. Carlton Fredericks to retort, "One wonders if the writer has ever pondered the discomfort and lack of aesthetic appeal of a colostomy bag."

In any case, one doesn't have to consume bran to obtain roughage. Whole grains of all kinds, plus most raw vegetables and fruits, are high in fiber. The foods that do so much for your health in what they supply the body are, so it seems, also good for you in the amount of residue that they leave over for the body to expel.

Garlic

This pungent plant occupies a cherished place in the history of folk medicine. It has been used as a disease preventive and all-around medicine since ancient times. Modern research has shown that the claims made so often in its behalf rest on much more than simple superstition. Experiments by reputable researchers published in reputable journals such as *The Lancet, Today's Health, Science Digest,* and *The German Medical Monthly* point up its possibilities in medical therapy.

Garlic, so it seems, can lower the blood pressure and also reduce cholesterol. It can strengthen the heart and prevent or retard hardening of the arteries. And it can function as an antibiotic in controlling many types of infection and disease.

Garlic, as we have already seen, contains sulfur and selenium, and at least the last-named mineral does have a cancer inhibiting effect. For that reason alone we should expect to find it on an anticancer food list. However, garlic also contains other substances that seem to curb cancer.

One of these substances is a bactericide called allicin. In 1957, two scientists at Western Reserve University isolated some allicin from garlic oil and gave it to mice that had been inoculated with cancer cells. None of the mice developed cancerous tumors. Another group of mice inoculated with similar cancer cells rapidly developed cancer and died.

The report on this seemingly important experiment was carried in the November 24, 1957, issue of *Science* magazine. A few months later another experiment was reported on the effect of garlic in treating cancer tumors in humans. The March-April 1958 issue of *Problems of Oncology* described the work of two Russian doctors who had found that garlic alleviated precancerous white spots on the lips. Its use in this regard was successful in 184 out of 194 patients tested. As a matter of fact, 166 of the patients needed only one application to get rid of these precancerous growths.

More recently, two Japanese scientists actually developed a cancer "vaccine" from garlic. The vaccine consisted of some tumor cells that they had exposed to an extract of fresh garlic. They then injected these cells into mice. When the mice subsequently received injections of millions of tumor cells, none of them developed cancer. Thus, the vaccine proved 100 percent effective, at least when it came to preventing mice from malignancy.

Unfortunately, like so many natural substances with confirmed anticarcinogenic properties, garlic has failed to excite any wide-spread interest in traditional Western medicine. It is, however, being used quite extensively by doctors in the Soviet Union for treating a variety of ills including flu, gout, rheumatism, and even kidney stones. Garlic, though not a staple of the regular Soviet diet, is very popular in the Southern Caucasus, a region that has become widely known for the number of its inhabitants who live to be well over one hundred.

Onions

Onions resemble garlic not only in their propensity to produce bad breath, but also in their ability to lower cholesterol and strengthen the heart. Along with garlic, they can control the rise in blood sugar in animals fed a high sugar diet. They may have an anticancer effect as well. Unfortunately, no research has been reported on this, so no one can say for sure. Nevertheless, anyone would be wise to include onions in his or her regular diet. They do contribute to human health.

Mushrooms

The mushroom is another plant that warrants our consideration and consumption. Mushrooms contain large amounts of important B vitamins, especially pantothenic acid. They also contain many useful minerals including iron, magnesium, calcium, copper, potassium, and phosphorus. According to a report by two Japanese scientists in the December 1966 issue of *Journal of Nutrition*, some species of mushrooms can significantly lower blood cholesterol levels. At least they have done so in rats who have been purposely fed a high-cholesterol diet.

More directly relevant for our purposes is the fact that many species of mushrooms contain specific antibiotic prop-

erties. Dr. William J. Robbins, working at the New York Bo-
tanical Gardens, found that 213 out of 332 kinds of mushrooms he examined contained substances that could destroy
harmful bacteria. One type of mushroom (*Boletus edulis*) has
been tested at the Sloan-Kettering Institute for Cancer Research and found to have a sharply inhibiting effect on induced tumors in mice.

Of course, not all mushrooms may prove so potent in
blocking cancer, and some may not contain antibiotic properties at all. However, their known richness in other ingredients important for human health, and their possibilities as
cancer deterrents, should give them a deserving place in our
daily diet.

Yogurt

Bulgaria traditionally has had a higher percentage of people
over 100 years of age than any other European country. In
Bulgaria, yogurt is a favorite foodstuff. Is there any connection?

Many have thought so. Such thoughts have been
strengthened in recent years by the discovery of three more
specific regions in the world where living beyond a hundred
is by no means a rarity. These areas are the already-
mentioned region of Southern Caucasus of the USSR, the
Hunza section of Pakistan, and the Vilcabamba Valley in
Ecuador. In at least the first two of these regions, yogurt or
some form of fermented milk is ingested quite regularly.

In the meantime some research has arisen which indicates that the prevalence of yogurt or yogurt-type foods in
these areas may not be a coincidence. Yogurt or other types
of fermented milk may well help human beings live longer
and live free of cancer.

As far back as 1932, the *Canadian Medical Association Journal* carried an article by a research physician named José M. Rosell. Dr. Rosell pointed out that fermented milks have often proved useful in treating many digestion problems. He wondered if it might not also prove helpful in handling many other types of diseases and disorders. Yogurt, he noted, contains lactic acid, and therefore it exhibits "demonstrated antiseptic powers."

More recent research has tended to bear him out. René Dubos, then of Rockefeller University, has shown that yogurt contains certain healthful bacteria that make laboratory animals more resistant to infection and to the aging process generally. A Vanderbilt University biochemist named George V. Mann has found that yogurt, if consumed in sufficient amounts, will lower cholesterol in the blood. (His experiments were done with human beings, first in Africa and then in the United States. In both cases, yogurt lowered cholesterol.)

At least two experiments have been reported showing that yogurt tends to be anticarcinogenic. One, reported by the National Cancer Institute, was conducted at the University of Nebraska. Three scientists infected two groups of mice with cancer cells. One group had received regularly a small amount of yogurt with their drinking water; the second had not. In the first group, more than a quarter of the tumor cells failed to grow as expected. In the control group all the cells grew. Concluded the scientists, "The above findings suggest that lactobacillic cultures synthesize components which have an anti-tumor effect."

Another experiment conducted in Europe showed even more striking results. An extract of *Lactobacillus*, such as is found in yogurt and buttermilk, was given to mice in whom cancers had been induced. Half of the mice not only stayed free of cancer, but became immune to any further cancers that were implanted in them.

This experiment was cited by three New York physicians in an article in the *Journal of the American Geriatric Society*. The physicians stressed the potential of yogurt and buttermilk in arresting or alleviating various health disorders. However, they noted that yogurt's antibiotic principle reaches its peak after forty-eight hours of growth and then gradually disappears over the next two weeks. To be most effective, therefore, yogurt should be consumed within two days after it is made.

The role of lactic acid in fermented milk opens up other possibilities for an anticancer dietary regimen. Apple cider vinegar also contains some lactic acid, and consequently its use by rural Vermonters as a folk medicine may not be without cause. It is also interesting to note that the people of the Southern Caucasus in the USSR eat much of their food pickled. Though pickling can sometimes cause cancer, as we saw in the case of China, it may also prevent it, depending on the way it is done. Food preserved in a lactic-acid-containing vinegar and free from injurious nitrites and fungus growths may actually strengthen our defenses against malignancy.

The Mighty Sardine

At the age of sixty-eight, the great German statesman Bismarck had settled into a decline that seemed destined to carry him to his deathbed. A lifetime of overindulging—overeating, overdrinking, oversmoking, and overworking—had finally caught up with him. His strength was failing fast.

But then Bismarck was introduced to a young Jewish physician named Schweninger who was reputed to have great abilities. Dr. Schweninger promptly put the Iron Chancellor on a diet consisting almost exclusively of herring. Says Bismarck's biographer A. J. P. Taylor, "However curious this seems by contemporary standards, it did the trick. Bismarck's weight went down . . . he slept long and peacefully; his eyes became clear, his skin fresh and almost youthful." According to Taylor, "Every observer noted the change in Bismarck; and it can be seen in his photographs. In 1877 he is bloated, choleric, bursting at the seams." In 1883, just before he met Schweninger, the photos showed "A bearded old man, bewildered at life and hardly able to control his twitchings long enough to face the camera. In 1885 he is fresh, clean-shaven, chin upright, face finely drawn, master of himself, seventy years old no doubt, but a man with a long life before him."

Bismarck then entered on the most productive era of his life. Of course, he did not stay on a diet of herring. His menu was later expanded to include, among other things, two raw eggs every day. He lived to a hale and hearty eighty-three years of age. If he had met Dr. Schweninger earlier, he probably would have lived much longer.

Herring, as we saw in the previous chapter, is a rich source of zinc, and this probably accounts, in part, for the transformation it wrought in the German chancellor. Herring, in company with many other seafoods, is also a source of selenium, calcium, and many other valuable minerals. But, perhaps the greatest nutriment to be derived from seafood in general, and from one particular kind of herring in general, is neither a vitamin nor a mineral. This is nucleic acid.

Essentially there are two kinds of nucleic acids, called RNA and DNA. They play a most crucial, but highly complex, role in the functioning of our cells. There is reason to believe that nourishing our cells with RNA nucleic acid by ingesting foods that contain substantial amounts of it can help us live longer, cancer-free lives.

The person who has pioneered the most in this area is a New York City physician named Benjamin S. Frank. He has evolved what he calls a "no-aging diet," which he claims can actually make people younger as well as cure many ailments. All this can be accomplished, he says, through nucleic acid accompanied by various vitamins.

The cardinal component in Dr. Frank's diet is the sardine. He favors sardines not only because they are rich in nucleic acid, but because they are also low in cholesterol. When one eats a sardine, one eats the whole organism. Frank's diet, therefore, called for the consumption of sardines four times a week. The smaller the sardine, the better it is, he says. Consequently Norwegian sardines are favored over American ones. But all sardines, which are forms of herring, are good.

He also favors other seafood such as salmon, lobster, shrimp, oysters, and other types of nonvertebrate sea animals. He recommends liver; beans such as lentils and pinto beans, and certain vegetables, including beets, asparagus, radishes, onions, scallions, mushrooms, spinach, cauliflower, and celery. All of these foods are, to a greater or lesser degree, fairly replete with nucleic acid or with substances that generate nucleic acid.

Does Dr. Frank's diet work? Virginia Castleton, beauty editor of *Prevention* magazine, gives it an enthusiastic endorsement. She has apparently tried it and found that it does work. A former colleague of mine also tried it, or at least a form of it. For about ten days he consumed a can of sardines every day plus forty tablets of brewer's yeast, which is also high in nucleic acid. At the end of this brief period his skin *seemed* to have taken on a fresher and more youthful texture, but such appearances can, of course, be deceiving.

Important support has come to Dr. Frank from a respected biochemist who has devoted most of his life to nucleic acid research. Professor Sheldon S. Hendler, Ph.D., chairman of the Division of Basic Sciences at the University of Baja California, calls *Dr. Frank's No-Aging Diet* (the title of the book in which Dr. Frank expounds his theory) "A significant landmark in the history of nutrition." Another biochemist, Dr. Hans J. Kugler, also applauds Frank's findings.

Will Dr. Frank's diet combat cancer? He claims that cancerous mice given injections of nucleic-acid-related nutrients plus other nutrient vitamins staged a complete recovery. "Tumors stopped growing, became smaller, then died. The mice lived on." He is careful not to claim that his diet will cure cancer in human beings. But the evidence does suggest that sardines, seafood in general, plus the other nucleic-acid-rich foodstuffs that he designates all deserve a place in our anticancer larder.

Asparagus

Some years ago a Pittsburgh dentist named Richard R. Vensel claimed he had cured himself of cancer of the eye as well as Hodgkin's disease (cancer of the lymph glands) by eating asparagus. Most medical practitioners, of course, ignored the claim, but one retired biochemist did not. Karl B. Lutz, also of Pittsburgh, began working with Vensel compiling case histories of those who had tried "asparagus therapy."

The cases, as Lutz reported them in a letter to *Prevention*, seemed almost astounding. One man who was completely incapacitated with a case of Hodgkin's disease was so fully recovered at the end of a year of asparagus therapy that doctors were unable to detect any sign of cancer. Another man, whose lung cancer was so far gone that surgeons refused to operate, cured himself in five months by eating asparagus. Other case histories recounted by Lutz are equally startling.

In the meantime, three organizations devoted to promoting the use of asparagus in treating cancer have sprung up. Their names and addresses, as given by *Let's Live* magazine in its February 1974 issue, are:

1. The International Association of Cancer Victims and Friends, Inc.
    155-d South Highway,
    Solana Beach, CA 92075
    (Manhattan Chapter: Box 1806, F.D.R. Station,
    New York, NY 10022)
2. Cancer Control Society
    2043 North Berendo
    Los Angeles, CA 90027
3. March of Truth on Cancer (information center only)
    P. O. Box 251
    Fort Belvoir, VA 22060

The first of these organizations, the International Association of Cancer Victims and Friends, Inc., maintains, in an information sheet, that "a group of sixty patients recovered their health taking the asparagus therapy. Patients began to feel better in two to four weeks. In this study it was found that all kinds of cancer responded, *except in those patients who had had mustard gas chemotherapy. It is not effective in those cases.*"

The group stresses that asparagus should never be consumed raw and should never be kept for more than a week. It is important to continue eating asparagus until a medical diagnosis shows the sufferer is cancer-free.

Is there any scientific basis for believing that asparagus works as these reports claim? Yes, there is. Lutz points out that asparagus is richly endowed with what are called histones. Science knows that human cells contain histones, along with enzymes and DNA. Histones seems to have something to do with a cell's functions, but scientists have as yet been unable to pinpoint what it is. Asparagus is also quite rich in folic acid—it is second only to liver in this respect—and it contains a fair amount of nucleic acid as well. So it is not beyond the limits of rational speculation that asparagus may have potent anticancer properties.

Lutz believes that all cancer patients should take four tablespoons of asparagus puree *twice daily*, morning and evening. The puree is made by simply dumping the contents of a can of asparagus into a blender and then liquifying it at a high speed. Since he, too, maintains that asparagus should be cooked before using, and since the two leading brands, Green Giant and Stokely, contain no preservatives, he says they may be used for this purpose.

What about asparagus as a cancer preventive? Lutz says that he and his wife each take two tablespoons of the puree, diluted with water to suit their taste, at both breakfast and dinner. And, he says, his most recent blood checkup showed substantial improvements over the last one.

The case for asparagus as a primary means for controlling cancer is certainly not proven by these claims. But since it is a health-building vegetable containing some anticarcinogenic nutrients, it too belongs on the anticancer menu.

Bounties from the Bees

During the 1930s a Russian biologist named Nicolai Tsitsin decided to survey Soviet citizens who had reached the age of 100 or more. He wrote to 200 such people and received about 150 replies. In going over their responses he was struck by one fact: An unusually high number of these centenarians were, or had been, beekeepers.

Now, longevity and freedom from cancer customarily go together. As further study has shown, this appears to be the case with beekeepers. One of France's most distinguished agricultural scientists, Alin Caillas—the recipient of the Grand Medal of Gold from the French Academy of Agriculture and a knight in the Legion of Honor—examined the amount of cancer among beekeepers in Europe. As expected, he found it to be almost nil. One study of the deaths of 1,000 beekeepers showed that only one of them had succumbed to cancer.

In this country, the Vermont physician D. C. Jarvis collaborated with New England's largest beekeeper, Charles Mraz of Middlebury, in a study of cancer incidence among beekeepers. In over two years of checking and rechecking, they were unable to find one beekeeper who had died of cancer. They did discover one man who had suffered from cancer of the lymph glands (Hodgkin's disease), but he had contracted the malady before he began keeping bees. What's more, after he began beekeeping, he became cured!

What is there about beekeeping that promoted such resistance to cancer? Beekeeping, to be sure, provides a healthful, outdoor existence, but so do many other occupations that do not confer such immunity to cancer. The answer would seem to lie in the fact that beekeepers, as a group, tend to consume more products from the bees than other groups.

These products are principally honey, which is well known, and pollen, which is much less well known. Let us see if these foods house any special factors that might help the human body fight cancer.

Honey has enjoyed a reputation as a health promoter since ancient times. Scientific investigation shows that such a reputation is warranted. Although a sweetening agent, the sugar in honey comes in a different form from that in the refined sugar that we customarily use. It consists largely of the types of sugar into which we have to convert table sugar before it can be assimilated. In other words, honey provides us with already converted sugar and thus spares the human body the task of having to carry out the conversion process itself. The bees, you see, have already done that job for us.

Honey contains other ingredients besides sugar. These include small amounts of various vitamins and minerals along with nine out of ten essential amino acids that build protein. You may recall that Dr. Henry Schroeder of the Dartmouth Medical School found that while white sugar tended to deplete chromium from the body, honey, along with dark brown sugar and molasses, tended to increase the body's store of this valuable trace mineral.

Honey apparently also contains other, heretofore unidentified, components that act as antibiotics. Back in the 1930s, Dr. W. G. Sackett, a bacteriologist with the Colorado Agriculture College, put various disease germs and other infectious bacteria into cultures of pure honey. All of these germs died, sometimes in as little as five hours. His tests were subsequently duplicated and substantiated by another bacteriologist, Dr. A. P. Sturtevant of the U.S. government's Bureau of Entomology.

More recently a British physician wrote in the *Journal of the American Medical Association* that he was using honey as an antiseptic. Said Dr. Robert Blomfield, "I have been using pure natural honey for the past few months in the accident and emergency departments where I work, and have found that, applied every two or three days under a dry dressing, it promotes the healing of ulcers and burns better than any other local applications I've used before."

Dr. Blomfield went on to say that honey "can be readily applied to any other surface wounds, including cuts and abrasions. And I can recommend it to all doctors as a very inexpensive and valuable cleansing and healing agent."

Many other uses have been made of the healing power of honey. For example, John Huber, a registered masseur in Eugene, Oregon, says that honey heals athlete's foot in four or five applications.

What is lacking are any specific tests to determine directly whether honey can deter cancer. However, the proven health benefits from honey, along with its proven role as a killer of harmful bacteria, plus the studies that show the rarity of cancer among beekeepers should convince most of us to substitute it for sugar whenever we can.

Though honey is the best-known bee product, it is not the only one. The beehive also produces another foodstuff that may well outrank honey as a promoter of longevity and as an immunizer against cancer. This is pollen.

Pollen is the male element of the flower and is brought back by the bees from their forays into the woods and fields. Professor Tsitsin felt that pollen played a greater role than honey itself in lengthening the life span of the beekeepers he studied, and he may very well have been right.

Pollen contains a good many vitamins, but it is especially rich in certain B vitamins such as B_3, pantothenic acid, and folic acid. It also includes many of the amino acids, some minerals (especially potassium), and rutin, a glucoside that has been found valuable in strengthening the walls of the capillaries. Furthermore, it contains minute amounts of hormones, which may explain why physicians at the University of Uppsala Medical School in Sweden have found it most effective in alleviating problems of the male prostate gland. (A nutrition-oriented physician of my acquaintance told me that he cured his own case of prostatitis by taking bee pollen tablets from Sweden.)

Pollen has also been used to help allergy sufferers. Dr. William G. Peterson, an Oklahoma allergist, says he recommends raw honey for his patients since honey, if it is unsifted and unheated, contains all the pollen, dust, and molds that cause 90 percent of all allergies.

Pollen has been found to be a splendid revitalizer. Consequently, it has become a favorite food for many athletes and their coaches. Steve Riddick, the crack American sprinter who won a gold medal during the Montreal Olympics of 1976, takes pollen tablets. "They're fantastic," he says. Tom McNab, who trained all of Britain's track and field athletes for the Olympics, says that at least 90 percent of them took pollen tablets daily. And, the Finnish Sporting Association actually supplies pollen tablets to the nation's top sports competitors. Says Finnish track coach Antli Lananaki, "Our studies show that it significantly improves their performance."

As with honey, we have no concrete evidence linking pollen specifically with cancer control. But, one project carried out at the Women's Clinic of the University of Vienna strongly suggests its value in this respect.

Dr. Peter Hernuss and six of his medical colleagues at the clinic had become disturbed by the possible side effects of radiotherapy and decided to see if pollen could not offset them. They were using radiotherapy to treat twenty-five women with cancer of the cervix that had advanced beyond the point where it could be treated by surgery. They began giving fifteen of the women three-quarters of an ounce of pollen three times a day. The other ten women received the same diet but without the pollen.

The results amazed Dr. Hernuss and his fellow physicians. Vitamin E levels in the pollen-receiving women went up 36 percent while they went *down* 43 percent in the control group. Vitamin C levels went down in both groups, but the pollen eaters suffered only one-third of the vitamin C decline of those who received no pollen. Cholesterol levels decreased in the pollen group, while they actually increased in the non-pollen group.

The concentration of red blood cells went up 4 percent in the pollen group but went down 12 percent in the nonpollen group. The colorless infection-fighting blood cells called the leukocytes did not decline anywhere near as much in the pollen group as they did in the nonpollen group. In many other medical tests, such as in the blood levels of certain enzymes, the pollen group fared significantly better than the nonpollen group.

As might be expected the fifteen women who received the pollen reported less than one-half as much bladder inflammation, less than one-third as much rectal inflammation, and about one-third as much general discomfort as the control group. Furthermore, they slept and ate much better.

All of these observations and tests, plus others too numerous for us to go into here, convinced Dr. Hernuss that "a favorable influence of the pollen diet as an adjutant to radiotherapy in female genital carcinoma was found." He called for further research into the working of what he termed "this natural curative agent."

The lessons for us are obvious. If we wish to enjoy the long, cancer free lives of most beekeepers, we should emulate their diet and eat honey and pollen.

Kelp

In olden times when an American Indian living along the coast became ill, he often ate seaweed. Modern science has shown that he was probably smart to do so. Research in this area is still limited, but it does indicate that seaweed possesses certain powers to protect us from health disorders, including at least certain types of cancer.

On the West Coast two University of California researchers, virologist E. Frank Deig and graduate student Douglas Ehresmann, have been experimenting with extracts from a red seaweed common to the waters of northern California. They have found that some varieties of this seaweed contain a substance that tends to block the activity of viruses. One ailment that it seems to alleviate is herpes simplex type II. This ailment produces sores in the genital area, and some experts believe it to be a cause of cervical cancer.

At Montreal's McGill University, meanwhile, researchers have found that another substance derived from seaweed, or kelp, can help protect the body from strontium 90. Strontium 90 is a radioactive gas that can cause cancer. In the opinion of some experts, it has become all too prevalent in our modern technological society. Whether or not this fear is justified, kelp contains a compound called sodium alginate, which helps the body to excrete strontium 90 before it can be absorbed.

Finally, you may recall the research reported in the preceding chapter indicating that iodine deficiencies may lead to breast cancer. Kelp, which is available in tablet form in health food stores, is an easy and inexpensive form of iodine, as was noted. It has its place in our anticancer diet.

Apples and Other Fruit

Apples, like so many other of the special foods we have examined in this chapter, occupy a special place in folklore. We have all heard the phrase "An apple a day keeps the doctor away." Interestingly enough, many other countries have similar sayings about the value of apples; and, again, interestingly enough, we find modern science vindicating and validating this folk belief.

Apples contain some vitamin C and potassium. More importantly, they contain a good deal of fiber to supply bulk for our bowels and help protect them from cancer. Still more importantly, apples contain generous amounts of a substance known as pectin.

Pectin is a gluey type of material that is indispensable for making jellies and jams. However, recent research has disclosed that pectin has much more to offer. Two California researchers fed eighteen volunteers daily amounts of pectin for a year and a half. All of the volunteers experienced a drop in blood cholesterol, although no other change was made in their diets.

Finally, and perhaps most importantly, pectin, like the sodium alginate found in kelp, may help to purge the system of strontium 90. At least it has this effect on laboratory animals. *Nature's Way* magazine reported in September 1976 that European scientists had found that when pectin was given to animals that had been given the radioactive gas, the pectin seemed to combine with the radioactive element in the gas, allowing the animals to excrete it harmlessly from their bodies. It is possible that pectin would have a similar effect on other serious, cancer-causing pollutants.

Apples probably constitute nature's best storehouse of pectin, but oranges, lemons, quinces, and currants also supply appreciable amounts. Actually, most fruits furnish at least some pectin. All of them provide some vitamins, some minerals, and some fiber. Therefore, you should put fruit in general and apples in particular on your anticancer list.

Ginseng

The root of ginseng, an extremely slow-growing plant—it takes six years to harvest a crop—has a long reputation as a restorer and general elixir. As with so many such folk remedies, science has given support to many of the claims made in its behalf. Tests conducted by qualified researchers in England, Switzerland, Bulgaria, Japan, and most of all in the Soviet Union, quite conclusively show that this root does tend to promote health and vitality. Indeed, some tests even show that it fosters mental ability, for Soviet telegraphers, after receiving ginseng, made far fewer errors than did the control group that received only a placebo.

As might be expected, ginseng also seems to have marked abilities to act against cancer. In research conducted at the Institute of Biologically Active Substances in Vladisvostok, USSR, ginseng has been found to inhibit the growth of various induced tumors in mice and rats, sometimes by as much as 48 percent. A Soviet test on humans also yielded encouraging results. Half of a group of lip cancer patients received a daily dose of ginseng; the other half did not. Both groups were then given radiotherapy. The group receiving the ginseng responded much better to the treatment. None of the ginseng receivers had relapses and in none of them did the cancer spread.

In this country Dr. Sungman Cha, a professor of biomedical sciences at Brown University, says that one day one of his associates happened to throw some ginseng extract into a culture medium containing cancer cells. To their surprise, the extract killed all the cells. Says Dr. Cha, "We finally determined that the cancer cells were . . . killed . . . by one of the panaxinols, a group of compounds found in ginseng. We don't know which of the panaxinols is responsible, but I do know it has a very potent effect on cancer cells grown in test tubes."

Of course, what kills cancer in a test tube may not do the same in the human body, but the findings of Dr. Cha and his associates, combined with the results of the Soviet studies, gives ginseng the right to be called an anticancer agent.

What about other herbs and cancer? Herbal medicine has traditionally regarded the juniper tree and the mandrake root as antidotes for cancer. However, no reliable evidence at all exists to indicate that they possess any anticarcinogenic powers. Modern science has isolated two agents from the periwinkle plant that tend to prolong the lives of cancer patients. These agents are now being marketed as drugs by Eli Lilly and Company (they are known as Velban and Oncovin). Furthermore, Dr. John Edwards of Connecticut, working under a grant from the National Cancer Institute, has found that certain chemical extracts from mountain laurel and bluebell, once concentrated and purified, will reduce the size of certain tumors in mice. There is undoubtedly a field here for some provocative and promising research.

Eggs

Strictly speaking, eggs do not properly belong in this chapter or even in this book. They have no known special properties that make them effective control agents for cancer. But eggs are such a healthful food and have been so falsely maligned that I could not end the chapter without discussing them.

Per capita egg consumption has gone down rather sharply in the United States since the 1950s, largely because of the cholesterol scare. Eggs are known to contain generous amounts of cholesterol; cholesterol is said to be conducive to heart problems; ergo, people should not eat eggs.

The conclusion seems logical enough. However, as one biologist once observed, nothing is more dangerous in biology than pure logic. That, as it turns out, is exactly the case with eggs and cholesterol.

To begin with, there is no absolute certainty that cholesterol in the blood produces or aggravates heart problems. Some studies do indicate such a relationship; other studies indicate quite the opposite. But be that as it may, *there is no solid evidence at all that the cholesterol in eggs increases cholesterol in the blood of human beings.* On the other hand there are several studies that indicate that it does not.

One of the studies was published in the December 1968 issue of the magazine *Metabolism*. Investigators at Highland Hospital in Oakland, California, fed thirteen people the equivalent of nine eggs a day each. Subsequent studies showed that of the thirteen, only two showed any appreciable increase in blood cholesterol, and these two had a history of problems in the cholesterol-cardiovascular area. Meanwhile, seven, or more than one-half of the group, actually showed *slightly lower* cholesterol levels at the end of the test period. Another, and more recent study done among students at UCLA showed the same results. Student volunteers instructed to eat eggs daily showed no higher cholesterol levels than those instructed to refrain from eggs during the test period.

Another interesting project that indicates that eggs far from being dangerous to the heart may actually protect it was done in Boston. A physician named Sam Berman put more than 400 overweight and middle-aged Boston policemen on a weight-reducing diet. As part of the diet, they were instructed to eat several eggs a day. *At the end of eight years none of these 400 middle-aged men had had a heart attack.*

Perhaps the most startling test was conducted by Doctors Aryler Hammond and Lawrence Garfinkel of the American Cancer Society. They surveyed the dietary habits of 800,409 persons over a six-year period. They divided the persons into two groups: those who ate five or more eggs a week and those who ate four or fewer eggs a week. The results: those who ate the most eggs experienced *fewer* deaths from heart attacks and strokes than those who ate lesser amounts of eggs.

More recently, the American Medical Association's own journal has published research that vindicates eggs and apparently all other cholesterol-rich foods as well. The October 25, 1976, issue of the AMA's journal reported the results of an intensive study conducted by four research physicians at the University of Michigan. The team of doctors carefully checked the eating habits of over four thousand adult residents in Tecumseh, Michigan. They found, to their amazement, that *the amount of cholesterol that a person consumes bears no relationship to the amount of cholesterol in that person's blood.* Since the subjects they studied came from widely diverse income, social, cultural, and ethnic backgrounds, they could be fairly judged as essentially representative of the average American population.

But even before this latest study came to light, a highly respected cardiologist had called attention to the many fallacies that for so long have clouded this question. This cardiologist is Mark D. Altschule, M.D., a visiting professor of medicine at Harvard University and a lecturer in medicine at Yale University.

Writing in *Executive Health* (vol. 10, no. 8), Dr. Altschule starts off by making the flat statement "Any real proof of a relation between cholesterol-fat dietary control on one hand and blood cholesterol levels and heart disease on the other hand is yet to be established." He then goes on to cite various animal studies that show no connection between the amount of cholesterol in the blood and heart and arterial problems. Seals, for example, suffer from a high incidence of atherosclerosis but have virtually no cholesterol. Baboons also develop heart attacks despite very low cholesterol levels.

Dr. Altschule then goes on to cite other research indicating that the same lack of relationship between blood cholesterol and heart problems exists in man. He notes that Trappist monks living on a very frugal vegetarian diet often, though not always, exhibit low cholesterol levels. Yet, these monks suffer heart attacks at the same rate as Benedictine monks who eat an ordinary diet.

The noted cardiologist then takes on the assertion that eating eggs or other cholesterol-rich foods will increase cholesterol in human beings, irrespective of whether such cholesterol is actually harmful. He points out that all the studies made that supposedly substantiate this claim were conducted on animals. More importantly, in all of them the cholesterol fed to the animals was not in the form in which cholesterol normally occurs in food. Instead it was given in a crystalline or powdered form usually prepared weeks in advance. *In this form* cholesterol, for various scientific reasons, which he cites, can damage the arterial wall.

Thus, says Dr. Altschule, it is not cholesterol feeding per se which has produced atherosclerosis in test animals. Their arterial problems resulted from the ingestion, usually in massive amounts, of *oxidized* cholesterol products which *do not normally occur in food.*"

The phrase "do not normally occur" needs some qualification. Cholesterol in the form of dried egg yolk, says Altschule, may present some problems, for it is an oxidized cholesterol product. Such dried egg yolk is used in many commercially prepared foods, such as cake mixes and dried soups. These are best avoided, he says. But eggs in their natural form, suggests the cardiologist, pose no peril.

Dr. Altschule's findings, presented here only in a summary form, further absolve eggs from any culpability in promoting heart disease or even high cholesterol. But, the exhaustive examination of egg eaters and non–egg eaters conducted by the American Cancer Society, along with the results of the weight-loss program conducted among Boston policemen, suggests something more. These two studies indicate that eggs may actually help protect the heart. Could such a supposition, so much at variance with the prevailing "wisdom," be true?

Yes, it could. For one thing eggs contain most of the minerals that guard the arteries and strengthen the heart. Secondly, and perhaps more importantly, eggs contain large amounts of a substance called lecithin (pronounced less'-a-thin). Several studies have been done concerning lecithin's possible role in preventing heart problems, and Dr. Charles E. Butterworth, professor of medicine at the University of

Alabama, in reviewing these studies, has accepted their basic findings. Lecithin, says this physician, does seem to help prevent heart ailments. (Dr. Butterworth is also the former chairman of the American Medical Association's Food and Nutrition Council. He was cited, you may recall, in chapter 3 in the discussion concerning how much vitamin C one should consume daily. As a matter of fact, his endorsement of lecithin came in the same article as the one in which he endorsed vitamin C.)

One last item concerning eggs may be of interest. The health magazine *Nature's Way* once reported the case of a sixty-three-year-old Australian who, because of throat problems, could eat nothing but raw eggs. As a result, he was consuming about seventy-two eggs a week. While this poor chap may have found his diet monotonous, he apparently did not find it harmful. Indeed, he said he felt fine. (Presumably, he was also taking some vitamin C supplementation since this vitamin is the one important nutrient that eggs lack.)[1]

Consequently, few people should have any qualms about eating eggs. The nutrients they contain, especially certain trace minerals, such as selenium, zinc, and chromium, should help keep us healthier and cancer-free. Those who worry about heart trouble, and the rest of us as well, would do well to avoid prepared foods containing dried egg yolks. But we now have expert opinion, backed up by a mass of evidence, that eggs in themselves do not endanger our hearts. Indeed, the evidence that now exists points to them as something of a protector for the heart.

---

[1]Both Dr. Vachon and I eat as many eggs as we wish. In his case this comes to five to seven eggs a week. In my case this amounts to between fifteen and twenty extra large eggs a week. Both of us have normal cholesterol, with my cholesterol count being somewhat lower than his.

7

Other Weapons, Other Ways

While diet may constitute our primary defense against cancer, we should not neglect other methods and means that can provide us with valuable protection. The time has now come to examine some of these other sources of cancer control.

Using Psychology to Prevent Cancer

The last book that supernutritionist J. I. Rodale penned before he died bore the title *Happy People Rarely Get Cancer*. As in so many other things that the elder Rodale wrote, he tended to let his ebullience and enthusiasm lead him into exaggeration. Happy people do get cancer. However, as in so much else that he wrote, Rodale was essentially on target. Happiness does seem to hinder the growth of malignant tumors.

This interesting relationship between cancer and personality was noted as far back as ancient Greece, when the physician Galen observed that melancholy women seemed to develop cancer much more frequently than optimistic women. In the nineteenth century a renown British physician, Sir James Paget, noted that "the cases are frequent in which deep anxiety, deferred hope and disappointment are quickly followed by the growth or increase of cancer. . . ." In the past few decades more rigorous research has tended to confirm and amplify such observations.

Let us start with an interesting animal experiment. Dr. Vernon Riley and his associates at the Pacific Northwest Research Foundation in Seattle wanted to see if stress would increase the cancer incidence among a strain of mice that was quite cancer-prone to begin with. Sure enough, they found that simply rotating the mice on a turntable was enough to increase their cancer rate.

They then put the mice in a highly restful setting, where they were shielded from the usual noise and other stresses and strains of the laboratory. Under normal laboratory conditions, eighty to a hundred percent of this particular strain of mice develop tumors eight to eighteen months after birth. But in their new, sheltered sanctuary, only 7 percent had developed cancer in fourteen months.

Do these experiments have any valid application to the study of cancer in human beings? An abundance of other studies indicates that they do.

Back in the 1950s, a psychologist named Lawrence LeShan examined the life histories of a group of cancer patients. He identified, so he said, a rather common pattern. Most of them as children had experienced a loss of either a parent or sibling, and this loss had impaired their ability to form close personal relationships. Later, as adolescents or young adults, they had achieved either a close personal relationship or a rewarding job only to have the relationship or the job abruptly terminated. These events left them feeling hopeless and lonely.

Another study done in the 1960s by Dr. William A. Greene, a psychiatrist at the University of Rochester, sheds further light on the possible role of psychology in cancer. Dr. Greene studied the life histories of three sets of twins. In each set, one twin had developed leukemia whereas the other had not. In each case Dr. Greene found that the twin who had contracted the malignancy had just gone through a period of psychological upheaval. In each case, the leukemia-free twin had not experienced such a stress. This led him to conclude that psychological stress might well be a major cause of cancer.

A European researcher has arrived at similar conclusions. Dr. H. J. F. Baltrusch of West Germany revealed to a cancer symposium in that country, the results of his study of more than 8,000 patients with different types of cancer. "In a majority of the patients," said Dr. Baltrusch, "clinical manifestations of malignancy occurred during a period of severe and intensive life stress frequently involving loss, separation, and other bereavements."

Stress, especially the stress produced by feelings of hopelessness and loss, thus emerges as a frequent factor in the development of cancer. But stress, of course, characterizes, to a greater or lesser degree, most of our lives. Additional research indicates, however, that stress, in and of itself, may not be as important as the manner in which we respond to it.

One very thorough study done by Dr. Caroline B. Thomas points this up. Dr. Thomas kept track of 1,337 medical students over a period of eighteen years. She found that those who developed cancer were likely to be quiet and nonaggressive people who generally suppressed, rather than expressed, their emotions and feelings. This study dovetails with another study done in England. There, Dr. Steven Greer surveyed 160 women who had been admitted to King's College Hospital in London with breast tumors. Some of the tumors were cancerous and some were not. Dr. Greer found that 60 percent of the women whose tumors were noncancerous were able to express their emotions fairly freely. Only one-third of the women whose tumors were malignant were able to do so. The other two-thirds of these women tended to bottle up their feelings.

In reviewing some of this research, Dr. Elizabeth M. Whelan draws the following conclusion: severe life stress may be important in bringing about a cancer, and so may be the way we handle that stress. The conclusions for those of us interested in preventing cancer should be reasonably obvious, though not necessarily easy to put into practice. We should first try to reduce the stress in our daily lives. This, of course, is often easier said than done. But there are ways of doing so. One frequent source of stress is simply the vast freedom we now enjoy. Modern man, especially the modern American, enjoys many more options than did his forebears. He can change jobs more easily, move more easily, marry and divorce more easily, and so on. Furthermore, his relative affluence confronts him with many more decisions to make, such as whether to spend his vacation at the seashore or in the mountains, whether to get this car or that car, whether to get this television set or that one.

Changes and frequent decision-making usually produce some stress. While we certainly do not want to give up the ability to make changes and choices, we should try to place limits on both. Developing some suitable routines—and I do not mean ruts—to govern the less vital areas of our existence can help greatly in lowering our daily degree of stress. Many people actually experience some stress in choosing the clothes they will wear for the day. A successful businessman I know has solved the problem easily. He has four winter suits and four summer suits. According to the season, he chooses one of the four suits in sequence and wears it for the week. Clothes for him have become a matter of routine.

More important, perhaps, than reducing the amount of stress in our lives—after all, as Dr. Hans Selye has noted, the complete absence of stress is death—is the development of ways of handling it. We should learn to find socially accept-able and personally agreeable ways of expressing our emo-tions; achieving true intimacy with one or more human be-ings may provide us with outlets for doing so. For some people, counseling or therapy may be helpful in breaking down the barriers they have erected around their own feel-ings. Religious observances and artistic pursuits also fre-quently furnish ways of channeling some of our feelings and frustrations outward.

A life of happiness and hope will never provide us with an iron-clad guarantee against cancer. But, it can probably turn the odds more in our favor. Diminishing the degree of stress in our daily existence, while developing better techniques for coping with the stress that does occur, can do much to further this end.

Using Psychology to Cure Cancer

My mother likes to tell the story of two women she knew who contracted cancer. One, when she heard the doctor's diag-nosis, promptly crawled into bed and stayed there until she died soon after. The other reacted with what might be called indignation. "Nonsense," she said and went right on living as if the cancer did not exist. She died many years later of natural causes.

A physician of my acquaintance, aware of my interest in this subject, once gave me an article to read from the old *Saturday Evening Post*. It was about a man who had been told that he had terminal cancer. However, his wife was pregnant at the time and he was eager to be present at the birth of his child. So he decided that he would try to stay alive until the baby was born. Twenty years later he was still alive and in good health.

Of course, such stories hardly constitute scientific evidence. In the case of the expectant father, part of the reason for his overcoming cancer may be attributed to what he ate. (Raw onion sandwiches were one of his favorite foods, and in his determination to defeat the doctor's diagnosis, he ate them religiously.) But they do suggest that a person who is determined to conquer cancer has a greatly improved chance of doing so.

Some physicians have begun to make use of such knowledge in helping their cancer patients recover. One of these is O. Carl Simonton, a former chief of radiation therapy at the U.S. Air Force's Medical Center at the Travis Air Force Base outside San Francisco. Dr. Simonton, who is now in private practice in Fort Worth, Texas, says the first patient he tried such techniques on was a sixty-one-year-old man whose throat cancer had become so severe that he could barely swallow his own saliva, let alone eat any food.

"I had him relax three times a day, mentally picture his disease, his treatment, and the way his body was interacting with the treatment and the disease. . . . I had him visualize an army of white blood cells coming, attacking and overcoming the cancer cells. The results of the treatment were both thrilling and frightening. Within two weeks his cancer had noticeably diminished and he was rapidly gaining weight. . . . The man had a complete remission."

Dr. Simonton says the results were frightening only because he had never witnessed such a turnaround. However, since then, he has had the satisfaction of seeing many such reversals and remissions. As he puts it, "You are more in charge of your life—and even the development and progress of a disease, such as cancer—than you may realize. You may actually, through a power within you, be able to decide whether you will live or die. . . ."

Dr. Simonton says that he has found that cancer patients often have a low self-image, have experienced a feeling of loss and hopelessness, have trouble venting their emotions, especially hostility, and frequently feel they have no reason for living. Working with his wife Stephanie, he seeks not so much to change the patient's personality as to further the patient's understanding of his problem and to help him realize that the question of his living or dying may, in many instances, be for the patient himself to decide. Those who wish to alter their outlook are given a cassette tape to play three times a day. The tape presents the recorded voice of Dr. Simonton telling them how to relax, how to picture the disease, and how to picture their body's conquest of it.

What the Simontons are doing may strike some as resembling faith healing, but that should not make anyone become suspicious. As it happens, faith healing is becoming increasingly accepted as one valid means of coping with cancer and other health disorders. More and more physicians and patients are using faith healing as an adjunct to other forms of cancer therapy. Says Dr. Lawrence LeShan, the psychologist who did one of the early studies linking cancer with personality, "The psychic healer is a specialist in mobilizing the patient's own resources." Dr. LeShan says he has seen, among other things, the regression of cancer through faith healing, and he has trained some 150 people, including 35 doctors, in faith healing methods.

A physician who read this book's chapter on Dr. Gerson when the book was still in manuscript offered the opinion that maybe it was Gerson's personality and not his diet that was responsible for his cures. In other words, maybe Gerson was achieving his results through psychological means. This, however, is most unlikely. Dr. Gerson was trained in the old school of German medicine and his manner was, if anything, somewhat brusque. Furthermore, he was so overworked that he actually was able to spend only a minimum of time with each patient. And, of course, it was his diet that he believed in and his diet that he stressed. Finally, he never gave his patients exaggerated hopes. He even told them that the odds were against them.

But Dr. Gerson and Dr. Simonton do have one thing in common. Both believed that the body itself could conquer cancer if it could mobilize sufficient resources to do so. A combination of dietary and psychological measures may someday succeed in stamping out much, if not most, of the country's incidence of fatal cancer.

Meditation

When transcendental meditation burst onto the American scene, most of us were prepared to shrug it off as simply another of the foolish fads that the sixties and the seventies seem to have spawned in profusion. The sight of its grand guru on television with his beard, robes, and cross-legged stance did little to dispel such an image. But then things began to change.

For one thing, it became apparent that the young people who were practicing transcendental meditation, or TM as it is called, were far from being hippies or hipsters. They wore ties and short hair, or dresses and long hair. This conservative appearance was buttressed by a pleasant and friendly demeanor. Perhaps there was something different, something worthwhile in TM.

Then came some studies carried out by, among others, some doctors at the Harvard Medical School. These studies showed that TM tended to produce several positive physiological changes in the human body. These included a lowering of the blood pressure, a lowering of the pulse beat, and a lowering of the blood lactate levels. This last-named phenomenon generally correlates fairly closely with a person's level of anxiety. Gradually, a substantial body of evidence emerged that showed that transcendental meditation combats the symptoms of stress and actually stress itself.

TM has gone on to win the enthusiastic endorsement of many medical practitioners, including Dr. Hans Selye, who is regarded by many as the world's greatest authority on stress. Since stress, as we have seen, does make a person more prone to cancer, TM deserves our careful consideration.

The practice of TM is really quite simple. A person sits in a comfortable chair and simply repeats to himself a meaningless word, called a mantra by TM's practitioners. The TM organization believes that this has to be a special word to suit the individual. But Dr. Herbert Benson, head of hypertension research at the Beth Israel Hospital in Boston, thinks differently. His research, he says, has shown that just about any word can be used providing it has no particular meaning to the meditator. (He has used the word *one* in his experiments.)

If you wish to take advantage of this stress reliever, then here is how to do it:

1. Make sure you have not eaten for at least two hours. Your stomach should be fairly empty before you try to meditate.
2. Sit in a comfortable chair, close your eyes, and think about anything you wish for about thirty seconds.
3. Then start to say the word *one* (or any other word that does not have any particular meaning to you) to yourself.
4. If you find your mind wandering, as you almost inevitably will, and you are forgetting to say the word, do not get upset. But when it seems convenient, return to repeating the word you have chosen.

5. When you have finished meditating, remain seated with your eyes closed and with your mind thinking about anything you wish to think about *for at least two minutes*. Failure to do this will actually make you irritable and may give you a headache.

Practitioners of TM, or relaxation response therapy as Dr. Benson calls it, usually find that they become more easygoing and happier in their everyday lives. They also frequently find that they possess more energy and need somewhat less sleep. Nearly everyone who has tried it (including the present writer) feels he or she has benefited from it.

An alternative to this do-it-yourself approach is to subscribe for a course at a TM center. You will have to pay about $120 and will attend about four sessions, including one with a teacher who will assign you a mantra and help you start to meditate. For many, this is probably a somewhat more effective way to begin, and if you can afford it, you should not hesitate to attend the sessions. But one way or another, any person concerned about cancer, regardless of his age or station, should try this simple technique. It won't make you into a different person, but it can calm you down and make it easier for you to get along with others as well as with yourself.

How long and how often should you meditate? The TM people say twenty minutes twice a day is the best schedule to follow. Dr. Benson seems to feel that a more flexible schedule could work just as well. However, two twenty-minute sessions, one before breakfast, the other before dinner, do seem to be a most useful way to take advantage of its benefits. At times it will seem that you can hardly meditate at all—for example, your mind may be filled with many tensions and problems. But don't let this distress you. Gradually, you will find yourself meditating better and better. One last suggestion: there is some indication that meditation goes better when people meditate together. So if you can join with one or more others for meditation sessions, so much the better.

Yoga

Transcendental meditation comes from India and bears some relationship with another well-known Hindu practice, yoga. As you may know, yoga consists of a series of breathing and body exercises. Do these exercises help alleviate stress? Some recent research indicates that they do.

A team of doctors at the Medical Institute of Benares Hindu University in India has made a three-year study of yoga. Interestingly enough, they really became interested in this ancient Hindu practice only after they saw how popular it was becoming in the Western world. None of them had ever practiced yoga before.

They found that yoga, especially if combined with meditation—actually most forms of yoga include some meditation—does yield substantial relief from a variety of stress diseases, including ulcers, insomnia, and high blood pressure. Furthermore, yoga made it easier for some people to shed excess weight or break long-standing drug habits. (Many Americans who have begun using TM have found that it has helped them stop smoking.)

The Indian doctors carried out their experiments not only on human subjects, including themselves, but on laboratory animals as well. They found, for example, that standing mice on their heads or placing them in other yoga postures enabled the animals to cope better with stressful situations.

Exercise

Yoga brings us to the question of exercise in general. There is no question that Western people, especially we Americans, place a rather extraordinary emphasis on exercise as a means of making people healthy. Indeed, we usually define physical fitness as the ability to run or jog a certain distance or to do a certain number of push-ups or to perform some similar physical feat. Although many, perhaps most, Americans do not engage in regular exercise, many of us zestfully swat tennis balls or golf balls or jog mile after mile in the belief that we are keeping ourselves hale and hearty.

The interesting aspect to all this is that no conclusive evidence exists to show that exercise actually improves a person's health. One study showed that while those who exercise regularly had about the same number of heart attacks as those who did not do so, the damage to their hearts was, on the average, somewhat less than that suffered by the average nonexerciser. This would seem, at first glance, to vindicate those who advocate exercise. We must always be wary of statistics, however, when they comprise a great number of other factors that have not been accounted for. For example, the exercise group most probably included a high proportion of people who did not smoke, did not drink, (at least not to excess), and who took care of themselves in other ways. The nonexercise group, on the other hand, probably included a disproportionately high number of people who did smoke, drink, and in other ways failed to take care of themselves. Viewed in this light, regular exercise may actually be seen as more harmful than helpful to health.

Actually a few doctors believe that most forms of exercise are actually dangerous to men over forty. And it must be said that professional athletes seem only rarely to live to advanced ages. I have come across the cases of ardent amateur tennis players who suffered heart attacks while still in their thirties. And I remember reading in a newspaper some time ago that the doctor who started the jogging craze had sustained a heart attack. From his hospital bed he was quoted as saying that he was reconsidering his advocacy of the sport.

   If exercise, as a means of promoting health and longevity, remains somewhat suspect, physical activity in a more natural form does appear to provide benefits in keeping us fit and free of cancer. The long-lived people who inhabit the Southern Caucasus of the USSR, the Hunza section of Pakistan, or the Vilcabamba Valley in Ecuador, all seem to keep busy at largely agricultural or domestic chores until they finally die. Thomas Paar, the most long-lived man in British history—he was born in 1483 and died in 1635—threshed grain and otherwise stayed physically active until his death at the age of 152. The British prime minister William Gladstone who lived to be eighty-nine liked to chop down trees. The British philosopher Bertrand Russell, who died in his nineties, was accustomed to walking several miles a day.

   The noted Harvard Law School dean Roscoe Pound, who wrote a five-volume work on American law between the ages of eighty-six and eighty-nine, was also a regular walker. During his later years he went on extensive walking trips through Europe. Alonzo Stagg still mowed his own lawn at the age of ninety-eight. Such long-lived presidents as John Adams, Thomas Jefferson, and James Madison busied themselves around their farms and plantations until they died. None of these men, it would be pointed out, died of cancer.

   Thus, while the value of strenuous exercise—especially when it is of a competitive nature—remains in doubt, the value of simpler forms of physical activity does seem to have proven itself. Our bodies were made to be used, and it is deeply regrettable that they are not used more often. Regularity rather than rigor seems to be the key factor in proper physical exertion, and simple walking may well be the most healthful exercise of all, at least for those who have passed their youth. A brisk daily walk, along with other forms of natural and noncompetitive physical activity, may do much to keep us healthy and cancer-free.

Mother's Milk and Cow's Milk

Some years ago, on a visit to Montreal, I picked up a copy of the French-Canadian health magazine *Prevenir*. Glancing through it, I noticed a letter from a physician who had treated numerous Quebec Indians, as well as numerous Quebec woodchoppers, in the northern part of the province. Cancer was unknown in the first group but quite common in the second.

This physician speculated that much of the difference may arise from the use, among nonnative Quebec citizens, of cow's milk to nourish infants. A substance created to feed a calf is not the same as one created to feed a baby, he observed, and he wondered whether or not the widespread substitition of cow's milk for mother's milk may not be a factor in the rising incidence of cancer generally. He mentioned that he had taken two maps of the world and colored in the areas on one of the maps where bottle feeding is common. On the other map, he had colored in the areas where cancer is common. The two maps, he pointed out, were virtually identical.

The physician noted that whenever he sought to discuss this issue with his colleagues or to show them his maps, they usually laughed at him. However, it is a safe bet that none of them are laughing anymore. We now have pretty solid evidence that bottle feeding creates vulnerability to cancer.

Mother's milk contains as much as six times the vitamin E of cow's milk, as well as twice the selenium. Mother's milk also has much more vitamin C. Furthermore, breast milk furnishes a rather rich supply of magnesium; pasteurized cow's milk supplies almost none. And breast milk is much lower in sodium (salt) than cow's milk. Finally, human milk contains a special vitamin-like nutrient that cow's milk lacks.

This nutrient may serve to modify the bacterial contents of a baby's intestinal tract.

There are still other differences between cow's milk, especially pasteurized cow's milk, and mother's milk; altogether they would seem to spell out a considerable difference in their respective effectiveness in nourishing a baby. Since many of the vitamins and minerals found much more abundantly in breast milk have also been found to have an anticarcinogenic effect, bottle feeding presumably can make a child into a more cancer-prone adult.

However, a new factor has entered the situation. Bottle feeding may increase not only the child's subsequent susceptibility to cancer but his mother's vulnerability to the disease as well. A study of 5,000 women conducted by the Cedars of Lebanon Hospital indicates that breast feeding is an ideal way to avoid breast cancer. The study found that no woman in the group who had nursed one child for as long as twelve months, or two children for as long as nine months each, had ever contracted breast cancer. The incidence of it among the other women in the group seemed to correlate generally with the amount of breast feeding they had done.

This study has, fortunately, aroused considerable attention in medical circles. It is probably one of the very few such studies cited in this book that your own physician is likely to have heard about. The lesson it has to teach is obvious. Any mother who wishes to reduce the chances that she will develop cancer should nurse her offspring. And in so doing, she will probably reduce the offspring's chances of eventually developing cancer as well.

Laetrile

In 1920 a California physician named Ernest T. Krebs claimed to have found a cure for cancer. His miracle medicine was simply an extract from apricot pits. However, the new drug, which he called Laetrile, turned out to be highly toxic. Consequently, no attempt was made to make or market it.

However, in 1952, Krebs's biochemist son, Ernest T. Krebs, Jr., announced that he had found a way to purify his father's discovery. This new form of Laetrile was safe for use. The question now arose as to whether it was at all effective.

The issue of Laetrile's ability to act against cancer gradually grew into a swirling, searing controversy. As the cancer rate climbed, more and more sufferers began desperately turning to Laetrile, looking upon it as their last hope for survival. At the same time, however, the full weight of the medical establishment came down on the side of its detractors. Laetrile, according to most medical and scientific organizations concerned with fighting cancer, was worthless. Those who believed in its efficacy were deluding themselves.

The theory behind Laetrile is that it releases hydrocyanic acid into the body. Normal cells can protect themselves against this acid but cancer cells cannot. Thus, the cancer cells are destroyed while the normal cells are preserved intact. (This last point is the key one. Modern medicine knows a number of ways to destroy cancer. The problem is to do so without killing the noncancer cells and thereby killing the patient.)

Is there any basis for believing in Laetrile? Certainly the case against it seems strong. It has been tested three times by the National Cancer Institute and at least four times by other health agencies. All of these tests, say spokesmen for the organizations that conducted them, failed to turn up any beneficial effects.

One study examined the case histories of twelve patients whom a Mexican physician claimed to have treated successfully with Laetrile. Indeed, the doctor, Ernesto Contreras, submitted them to the Food and Drug Administration and the National Cancer Institute as the most spectacular of his success stories. But of the nine patients whose records the FDA and the institute could obtain and review, six had succumbed to cancer; one still had cancer, which had spread since the Laetrile treatments; one had also used conventional medical therapy; and the ninth had died of another disease. This would scarcely seem to be an impressive record of success.

But the backers of Laetrile are not without arguments to support their views. First, the Food and Drug Administration had resolutely refused to test the drug on human beings. Various attempts by various pro-Laetrile organizations to conduct such tests themselves had met firm FDA rejection. Furthermore, a certain amount of dissension had arisen regarding the Laetrile tests that the National Cancer Institute has run on animals. Dr. Dean Burke, a biochemist who headed the institute's cytochemistry division resigned over this point. He maintained that the tests, properly interpreted, show Laetrile to have a deterrent effect on cancer.

Some other data also tend to give aid and comfort to Laetrile's supporters. Although many areas in the world have little cancer, only one area is completely cancer-free. This area, according to a United Nations study, is the Hunza region of Pakistan. As it happens, this is also the only region that makes apricot pits an integral part of its regular diet. An oil extracted from the pits constitutes the Hunza people's main cooking oil.

In this country, the Pueblo Indians of Taos, New Mexico, consume a beverage made from the pits of apricots, peaches, and cherries. They enjoy an exceptionally low rate of cancer. Robert G. Houston, a writer who was doing cancer research among these Indians, began drinking blender shakes made from their recipe. He told *Prevention* that on his third day of drinking such shakes, two benign skin growths on his arm began to shrivel up. By the seventh day, they were completely gone. Houston adds that two of his friends who began drinking the shakes had the same experience.

Finally, an Israeli physician, Dr. David Rubin of the Hebrew University Medical School, began in 1977 a controlled study involving twenty patients with advanced breast cancer. None of the women were expected to live more than six months. Ten of them were receiving Laetrile injections while the other ten were receiving a placebo. As this is being written, the study is still underway and the final results are not in. But in a telephone interview with an American newspaper in May 1977, Dr. Rubin revealed one preliminary finding. Most of the women receiving Laetrile did not complain of pain; most of those receiving placebos did complain of pain.

Some doctors in this country, as well as in Mexico and Canada, where the sale and use of Laetrile is legal, claim that the drug does work, at least on some patients. Dr. Stewart Jones of Palo Alto, California, says he saved his own mother from death through the administration of Laetrile. And interesting incidents keep cropping up that seem to support those who argue in Laetrile's behalf. For example, four-year-old Robbie Medwar of Wilbraham, Massachusetts, was diagnosed in September 1976 as suffering from a growth on the base of his spine. The growth (esonophilic granuloma) was nonmalignant but was potentially as deadly as cancer. Robbie's mother, a registered nurse, rejected her doctor's recommendation for radiation and surgery. Instead, she gave the youngster small amounts of Laetrile daily. By November, X rays showed no sign of the growth.

What shall we make of all this mass of conflicting evidence? A few conclusions can be drawn. Firstly, Laetrile probably does no one any harm. Even some of its fiercest opponents do not claim that it can do any damage to the human body. Secondly, Laetrile, while it probably does not provide the world with a sweeping solution to its cancer problem, may help some people overcome the disease. Thirdly, Laetrile, as we have seen, is the proprietary name for a substance found in apricot pits. But this substance, which is chemically identified as nitriloside, can be found in many other foods. What's more, these nitriloside-bearing foods have many better-proven health-giving properties as well.

Food rich in Laetrile-like nitrilosides include many fruits, such as apples, cherries, cranberries, prunes, plums, pears, lemons, and limes, in addition, of course, to apricots. They also include many legumes, such as kidney beans, chick-peas, and lentils; and many whole grains, such as millet and buckwheat. Almonds, sweet potatoes, lettuce, and linseed have also been identified as nitriloside sources. Sorghum contains quite a bit of nitriloside, although molasses, which is like sorghum and which is rich in many minerals and vitamins, contains none.

Some qualifications must be appended to this list. For one thing, the fruits must be eaten whole, the kernels or seeds included. Also, sweet potatoes and lettuce grown in America or Europe may no longer contain any nitriloside. Finally, the legumes and grains mentioned are highest in nitriloside content when they are in the sprouting stage. Mung bean sprouts and alfalfa sprouts supply especially large amounts of this possibly anticarcinogenic substance.

Keeping these facts in mind, you would do well to partake heavily and heartily of these nitriloside-containing foods. Even if their nitrilosides turn out to be worthless in combating cancer, as well they may, you will still be gaining many other nutrients that promote better health and increased resistance to malignancy.

"A Checkup and a Check"

Most of us are familiar with the oft-broadcast slogan of the American Cancer Society asserting that the way to fight cancer is by having frequent checkups and by making frequent financial contributions to the society. How effective are these two methods of combating cancer?

As far as medical checkups go, while they may do some good in certain cases, more and more evidence is piling up that they are of limited effectiveness at best. For example, Dr. Katherine Boucot and some associates at the Medical College of Pennsylvania decided to see if they could increase the low rate of recovery from lung cancer through more frequent checkups. They gave 6,136 males over the age of forty-five chest X rays every six months for ten years. Over the course of this period, 121 of the group were found to have lung cancer and were given immediate and sustained treatment. But only 8 percent of them survived five years. Since this is the same survival rate for lung cancer patients who have come to the doctor only when actual symptoms have started to appear, the checkup program can hardly be deemed a success.

In another study, Dr. Charles Moertel surveyed the results of regular rectal examinations to detect rectal cancer. Of the 42,207 patients examined, only 55 were found to have any malignancy. Dr. Moertel concluded that "the truly routine proctoscopic evaluation does not seem to be a practical screening test."

Another cancer detection method that has come to the fore in recent years is mammography. It is considered quite effective in spotting early signs of breast cancer. However, in this case, the detection may not only discover the disease, but also help develop it. Mammography involves X-raying the breast, and the X rays themselves can cause cancer. Because of this danger, many medical experts now recommend regular mammography examinations only for women who are over fifty-five and women whose family histories show a record of susceptibility to breast cancer.

Then there is the pap smear, which does seem to offer a high degree of accuracy and sensitivity in the early diagnosis of cancer of the uterine cervix. Its supporters point to the fact that the death rates from this form of cancer have gone down quite dramatically since this detection device came on the scene in the 1950s. However, a Canadian study has shown that the decline in the death rate from this form of cancer in the province of British Columbia, where 80 percent of the women inhabitants took the test, was about the same as the decline in the province of Ontario, where only 20 percent of the women took the test.

In the United States, some have pointed to the 50 percent decrease in death from cervical cancer between 1930 and 1966 as proof of the test's efficaciousness. But it seems that half of the decline took place before the pap smear began to achieve widespread acceptance and use. Some have rather unkindly, but not unknowingly, observed that though the test is often useful, another and perhaps equally valid factor in the reduction in cervical cancer mortality has been the rising number of unnecessary hysterectomies performed on American women during this time.

In surveying such studies as these, as well as the results of regular checkups in the detection and cure of other medical ailments, Dr. Richard Spark of the Harvard Medical School has concluded that, in general, such routine checkups have little protective value. "As unpleasant as it may sound to those who would like to believe otherwise," says Dr. Spark, "most diseases can be detected only after symptoms appear. Furthermore, with the exception of hypertension [high blood pressure] there is no convincing evidence that treatment of diseases before the onset of symptoms offers any long-term advantage over treatment that is initiated after symptoms appear." Dr. Spark does regard pap smears as useful devices for detecting uterine cancer. He also sees utility in tests for hypertension. But otherwise, he says, "repetitive annual exams of healthy individuals seem to be profitable only for the physician."

8

What Killed
Adelle Davis?

The Bible tells us that by the fruit of the tree we shall know what type it is. A more modern saying maintains that the proof of the pudding is in the eating. These adages conform to the criteria of both modern science and common sense. As science puts it, theories, to be valid, must be in accord with the facts. As common sense puts it, theories, to be valid, must work.

Over the course of recent decades several so-called supernutritionists have gained the public spotlight by promoting and observing, to a greater or lesser degree, many of the dietary rules that we have been examining. How have they fared?

In general most of the supernutritionists have fared very well. They have, for the most part, enjoyed long and cancer-free lives. In many cases, they have also demonstrated remarkable vitality and vigor in their later years. The late Bernarr MacFadden, for instance, parachuted from a plane on his eighty-third birthday, while the still-living Gaylord Hauser embarked on a worldwide lecture tour at the age of eighty. A lesser-known supernutritionist, Winfield Franklin of Warren, New Jersey, celebrated his seventy-fifth birthday in 1973 by running a full seventy-five miles. (He circled his local high school track field 300 times in nine hours and forty-five minutes.)

Of course, some supernutritionists have not lived to advanced ages. But we should bear in mind that many people are attracted to the nutrition field by their existing health problems. One example of this is J. I. Rodale, who died of heart failure at the age of seventy-two. Rodale suffered from a heart murmur from infancy. Furthermore, his father and most of his brothers died before reaching the age of sixty. Rodale's attention to diet and physical activity—he was a great believer in walking—probably lengthened his life by fifteen years or more. And, he, like the others, never contracted cancer.

But one glaring exception stands out: Adelle Davis, who died of cancer in 1974 at the age of seventy.

Adelle was an ardent advocate of many of the nutrients that, we have seen, tend to prevent, and possibly even cure cancer. She took goodly amounts of vitamin A, vitamin E, magnesium, and other apparently anticarcinogenic food substances every day. Does this mean that these substances are without value in cancer control? Or are there other reasons to explain her death?

Adelle—and so infectious was her enthusiasm for her cause that most of us who never knew her still tend to refer to her by her first name—offered another reason for what happened. She blamed it on overexposure to X rays. As she told her close friend and confidante, Betty Lee Morales, she was revising her books when her publishers decided to take out a life insurance policy on her. They were concerned as to what might happen if she were to die before the revisions were completed.

Such life insurance policies are rather common in the business world and Adelle agreed to go for the necessary examinations. These examinations included, she said, a large number of X rays. We can well believe her on this point, for hospitals these days, concerned about meeting their rising costs in the face of their growing numbers of empty beds, have begun taking extra amounts of X rays as one way of making extra money.

A few days after she completed the tests, she received a call from the examining physician. The X rays had, for some reason or another, not turned out clearly. There had been a foul-up. Would she come back for a second batch?

She consented and again found herself being X-rayed all over. They must have shot dozens, she said. "Tracing it back, I realize now I have never felt well another day since then."

That the X rays could have contributed to the cancer that two years later would take her life seems most plausible. Adelle died of bone cancer, and this form of malignancy frequently results from radiation. Furthermore, we know that the cancer appeared soon after the X rays were taken, although the X rays themselves showed her to be free of malignancy. The examining physician even congratulated her on her fine physical condition.

However X rays, when they do cause cancer, rarely, if ever, cause it so rapidly. Almost always the malignancy occurs only some time later. Furthermore, Miss Davis was not, we had all assumed, an ordinary person. Her emphasis on nutrition and her ingestion of so many of the food substances that fight cancer impels us to seek for further reasons behind her tragic death.

Ms. Morales provides some other clues to what these

might be. Up until the time she contracted cancer, Adelle Davis smoked two packs of cigarettes a day. (This probably explains why her books fail to discuss the role of cigarette smoking in health disorders.) What's more, she went through a period of alcoholism after her divorce from her first husband. She subsequently underwent extensive psychotherapy, which included, under careful supervision by a psychiatrist, the taking of LSD. Some years ago a book entitled *Explorations of Inner Space* appeared on the stands. The author's name was given as Jane Dunbar. Actually, Jane Dunbar was Adelle Davis writing under a pseudonym.

Obviously, none of these experiences, especially the cigarette smoking, did her health any good. But more important perhaps than the physical harm that the cigarettes, the alcohol, and the LSD caused was the severe stress that they signaled. Adelle Davis, so it seems, led a hectic and somewhat harrowing existence, frequently feeling the hopelessness and sense of loss that, as we have seen, so often characterize cancer patients at previous stages of their lives. In some respects, she almost seems to have been a psychological prototype of the kind of person who most frequently develops cancer.

If Adelle Davis may have had, to some degree, a psychological disposition to develop cancer, her diet may not have defended her from malignancy as she so optimistically supposed. A careful analysis indicates that it contained deficiencies that may have offset many of its more protective elements. Indeed, in some respects, some of her dietary practices may have even been conducive to cancer.

To begin with, while Adelle believed that vitamin C could counteract many forms of infection and disease, she also believed that sufficient vitamin C could be obtained from regular food sources. Thus, she apparently took no vitamin C supplementation on a regular basis. Since research, which we have already reviewed, points to heavy doses of vitamin C as possibly the single best means for curbing cancer, Adelle, in this respect, may have erred on the side of underestimating the need for high vitamin dosages.

For her, this was especially important, given some of the other aspects of her life. Smoking is believed to drain vitamin C from the body, and the two packs a day that she smoked for so long must have robbed her of much of the vitamin C she was obtaining from her regular diet. A still greater source of vitamin C depletion in the body, however, is stress. Dr. Klenner estimates that just a few brief moments of anger, for example, can consume several thousand milligrams of the vitamin, if the angry person has that much in him. Animals that manufacture their own vitamin C manufacture many times more of it when placed under stress conditions. Given the ups and downs of Adelle's life, with its frequent work as well as emotional pressure, one can speculate that she was obtaining far less vitamin C than she needed.

Then there is the question of brewer's yeast. As anyone who has read her works knows, this was one of Adelle Davis's favorite food supplements. But, during most of the time that she lived and wrote, food manufacturers had not learned how, or simply had not bothered, to remove the bitterness from brewer's yeast. This led her to recommend the use of torula yeast, which is substantially less bitter. However, though less bitter, torula yeast is also far less nourishing. It contains no selenium and nowhere near as much chromium as brewer's yeast. And it may be deficient in other ways as well. (Most of the material on the role of these important trace elements was only starting to come out at the time of Adelle Davis's death.)

But these may not be the most important deficiencies in the Davis diet. Two potentially more major misconceptions deal with her approach to protein and fat. These deserve more careful and detailed consideration.

Fats

Adelle Davis took a rather tolerant attitude toward fats. True, she felt that the doubling of American fat consumption in her lifetime had aggravated many of the nation's health problems. Yet, she also warned continuously of the dangers that she believed arose from eating too little fat. "Persons who intentionally restrict their fat intake probably get too little of the essential fatty acids to sustain health," she once observed.

Adelle noted that high fat levels in the blood do make a person more susceptible to heart attacks, but she maintained that low-fat diets could also do heart patients injury. For most people, she felt, fat intake should pose no problems. "Fats are needed to improve the flavor of foods, to satisfy the appetite, and to stimulate bile flow," she pointed out in one of her last books, *Let's Get Well*. "Butter, cream, gravies, rich cheeses, and other natural fats rarely need to be restricted, provided weight permits and the diet includes all nutrients that assure adequate absorption and utilization," she somewhat blithely added.

In one of her earlier books she actually seemed to encourage increased consumption of fats, for she said that "eating too little fat is probably a major cause of overweight," one reason being that "fats are more satisfying than are any other foods." If Adelle practiced what she preached in this regard, she may have made herself more vulnerable to cancer.

For one thing, a high fat intake causes the body to excrete magnesium, and magnesium, as we saw earlier, constitutes one of our major mineral defenders against cancer. Much more important, however, is the impact that fat consumption can create on the body's hormonal balance. Research revealed at a National Cancer Institute conference in 1975, one year after Adelle's death, shows that fat may alter the pattern of hormone production in the body, increasing the amount of hormones that cause cancer.

The conference was held in May of 1975, but its proceedings and findings were not reported until December. The research on fats and cancer was disclosed by Dr. John Berg of the University of Iowa. Dr. Berg told the conferees that fats, especially animal fats, tend to stimulate the body's hormonal system "producing the same effect that one would obtain running a diesel engine on high-octane airplane fuel." He pointed out that countries with a high fat consumption have five to ten times as much breast cancer, for example, as those with low fat consumption.

Although Dr. Berg pointed to animal fats, which fall into the category of saturated fats, as the major culprit in cancer creation, other evidence indicates that polyunsaturated fats may, under certain conditions, prove even more carcinogenic.

The eye-opening event that first brought this fact to light was a study conducted from 1959 to 1964 at a veteran's hospital in Los Angeles. Some 422 patients were put on a diet that was high in polyunsaturated fats, such as vegetable oils, and low in saturated fats, such as are found in meat, butter, cream, and so on. An almost equal number, 424, ate what was called the "standard American diet." Those who ate the diet high in polyunsaturates experienced a lower death rate from heart attacks during the ten-year period. (There were forty-eight such deaths in this group compared to seventy in the group consuming the standard American diet.) But when the doctors conducting the study rechecked their results, they found that the polyunsaturate group suffered a much higher death rate from cancer, *The net result was a death rate for both groups that was almost the same.*

Three years later, Dr. Denham Harman of the University of Nebraska reported on experiments with female mice in which he increased their incidence of tumors through feeding them unsaturated fats. He also foreshadowed and, at the same time, amplified, the subsequent findings of Dr. Berg by noting that in twenty-three countries he surveyed he had found a distinct relationship between the consumption of fats and oils and the death rate from several kinds of cancer in persons over fifty-five years of age.

This same year, the magazine *Nutrition Today* disclosed an experiment which can send chills up and down the spine of a person who has been conscientiously consuming polyunsaturates in the desire to lower his cholesterol. A group of laboratory animals were fed heated corn oil, while another group was fed heated butter over a forty-month period. Those who received the corn oil, which is a polyunsaturate recommended by many doctors to patients with high cholesterol, tended to develop diarrhea and rough fur and showed lower growth rates. Furthermore, *every single one of these animals developed tumors.* This directly contrasted with what happened to the animals receiving the heated butter. Not one member of this group developed tumors.

This experiment by no means negates the findings of Dr. Berg and others that saturated fats can cause cancer. What it does suggest is that polyunsaturates can be even more dangerous.

Dr. Mark D. Altschule, the Harvard-Yale cardiologist whose report on eggs was cited in the previous chapter, underscores the many perils that polyunsaturates can pose to the human body. He points out that corn oil, *even when unheated,* can, in very large amounts, prove poisonous to rabbits and rats. Excessive intake of polyunsaturates has also caused infants to become severely anemic and has made their bodies swell because of a marked retention of water in the tissues. "What happens", says Dr. Altschule, "is that the excessive unsaturated fatty acid intake greatly disturbs the vitamin E balance in the body and leads to vitamin E deficiency, and the anemia is actually a vitamin E deficiency anemia."

Altschule also takes note of the studies linking unsaturates to cancer and then goes on to cite an interesting piece of research regarding polyunsaturates and aging. This study sharply connected high consumption of polyunsaturates with signs of premature aging such as wrinkles, skin looseness, and so on. Some 78 percent of those studied who had been deliberately following a diet high in polyunsaturates showed such signs of advanced age. (Dr. Denham Harman has found that the life span of mice would be shortened as the amount and/or degree of unsaturation of their dietary fat was increased.)

Cardiologist Altschule even voices disbelief that such fats offer any protection against heart problems. He quotes an editorial in the *American Heart Journal* as saying "It is known that polyunsaturates have increased in the average American diet almost three-fold over the past three decades *without the slightest decrease in heart disease mortality*—which result logically could be expected to follow if this food did, in fact, exert a positive clinical effect." (Italics were added by Altschule. For our purposes, it is interesting to observe that this increased intake of unsaturates was accompanied by a steady spiraling of the nation's cancer rate.)

Dr. Altschule goes on to pinpoint one research study that should alert all those who use margarine in the belief that they are helping their hearts. Margarine makers, so it seems, use a production process that converts a large percentage of their product's unsaturated fats into a different form. And feeding test animals with this form of unsaturate—it is known as the "trans" form—actually raised the animals' cholesterol levels and increased their incidence of arterial damage!

Obviously, then, polyunsaturates should be consumed with care. Firstly, we should make sure that they are not rancid for rancid vegetable fats produce a potent cancer-causing substance called malonaldehyde. Secondly, we further. In studying a group of vegetarian women, Dr. Bruce K. Armstrong of the University of Western Australia found should avoid using them for cooking as much as possible. (Butter, or even olive oil, which is what is called a monosaturate, are better for this purpose.) Thirdly, we should take vitamin E for this vitamin offers us some protection from pernicious peroxides that such fats can produce in our bodies. It is these peroxides that are believed responsible for the link between such fats and cancer. Even such a conservative nutritionist as Jean Mayer believes that a diet high in polyunsaturates can benefit from vitamin E supplementation.

But, you may be wondering, why not simply eliminate the unsaturates altogether from our diet? This, first of all, is not feasible for most of us. Then, polyunsaturates, cautiously consumed, do have a distinct role to play in human health. They are good providers of certain acids that the human body needs. Finally, we should remember that saturated fats can also cause cancer.

An interesting experiment reported by researchers at the Boston University Medical School in May 1977 may serve to sum up this rather lengthy examination of the role of fats in cancer and well-being. Three different groups of rats received injections of a chemical (OMH) known to cause bowel cancer. One of the animal groups was fed a diet high in vegetable or unsaturated fats; the second group was nourished on a diet high in animal or saturated fats; and a third group was given a diet low in all kinds of fats.

The results? All of those receiving the diet high in vegetable fats contracted cancer of the colon. Some 85 percent of those receiving the diet high in saturated fats developed cancer. But of those fed the diet low in both types of fats, only 50 percent came down with cancer. Thus a low fat diet apparently enabled one-half of a group of exposed rats to escape malignancy.

There would appear to be an important lesson here for all of us who are concerned about cancer. It is tragic that

Adelle Davis did not live long enough to learn it. But hopefully her many admirers and fans, of whom the present writer is one, will do so.

Protein

If Adelle Davis tended to look with indulgence on fats, she positively glowed with pleasure at protein. She scoffed at the Food and Nutrition Board's recommended daily allowance of 54 grams for men and 46 for women, claiming it was far too low. "If you wish to maintain your attractiveness, vigor, and youthfulness as long as is humanly possible, it is probably wise to eat considerably more protein than the Board recommends," she once wrote. For people whose diet may have been deficient for some time, she urged the consumption of 150 or more grams a day for a month or more. For Adelle Davis, protein apparently could do no wrong.

Miss Davis, as one might suppose, also believed that protein could help to combat cancer. In this she was joined, oddly enough, by her foremost antagonist, Jean Mayer. Although Dr. Mayer so disliked Adelle Davis that he customarily disdained to call her by name—"a pop lady nutritionist" was the phrase he customarily used to refer to her—he seems to have agreed with her on this point. Mayer has said that cancer patients should take care to consume enough protein.

Unanimity between two such diverse nutritionists on this point would seem to clinch the case for protein. But does it? Let us, in Al Smith's famous phrase, look at the record.

There have been some animal experiments to test this theory. They have produced rather mixed results. Some of them—and these are the ones that Adelle cited—indicate that protein could have an inhibiting effect on cancer. Others, however, indicate the opposite.

When it comes to humans, however, the evidence is much less mixed. Generally it points to high protein consumption as having a causative rather than a curative effect on the development of malignancy.

To begin with, we have the cause of Dr. Gerson. As you will recall, he placed his patients on diets that were almost devoid of protein. It is difficult to imagine that he would have scored so many successes if protein had had the reverse effect of what he intended.

As we look around the world we find that low- rather than high-protein diets tend to correlate with reduced cancer incidence, as well as with longer life. Take those three regions that are known for their large numbers of centenarians and their remarkable freedom from cancer, the Southern Caucasus of the USSR, the Hunza section of Pakistan, and the Vilcabamba Valley in Ecuador. Dr. Alexander Leaf of Massachusetts General Hospital visited all three regions in 1973 and found protein consumption quite low in two of them. The Hunzas consumed about fifty protein grams a day, he estimated, while the Ecuadorian group ingested only thirty-five to thirty-eight grams.

In the Soviet region he studied, protein consumption, so he believed, reached seventy to ninety grams a day. However, his estimates here may be a bit off, for other observers seem to report a somewhat lower protein intake. In any case, this is still somewhat below the average American protein consumption. Furthermore, it is interesting to note that most of the protein came not from meat but from vegetable and dairy sources.

In the West, observers have long noted the longevity of vegetarians whose diets usually of necessity fall somewhat short in protein. Thomas Paar, the Englishman who lived 152 years, was a vegetarian. So were George Bernard Shaw, Bernarr MacFadden, and many other more notable personages who achieved a lengthy life span. They also remained free of cancer. Furthermore, American blacks generally eat less protein than American whites. Though their diets are often poor in other respects, and though they suffer more heavily from other health disorders, blacks enjoy an appreciably lower cancer rate.

However, the most definitive American study done on this point compared the cancer rates of Seventh Day Adventists with those of Mormons. Both religious groups frown on smoking and alcohol, and both promote and pursue a basically identical life-style. There is, however, one important difference. Seventh Day Adventists do not generally eat meat; Mormons do.

At a 1975 symposium on nutrition and cancer, Dr. Roland Phillips of Loma Linda University presented some carefully done research covering the respective cancer rates of these two religious groups. The essential conclusion was that the non-meat-eating Seventh Day Adventists experience a much lower cancer rate than do the meat-eating Mormons. What makes this finding even more determinative is the fact that the Mormons are heavily concentrated in Utah, which is a high-selenium state. As you will remember from our previous examination of this trace mineral, its presence in the soil in appreciable amounts almost always signals a low cancer rate. And to be sure, Utah does have a comparatively low incidence of cancer. But despite this fortuitous factor, Mormons still contract cancer more often than do Seventh Day Adventists.

As if this wasn't enough to indict meat, some further study came up with still more telling evidence. This subsequent study found that those converted Seventh Day Adventists who had once eaten meat ran a risk of developing cancer that, while comparatively small in relation to the American average, was nevertheless two to three times greater than those who had been vegetarians all their lives.

Other research tends to validate these findings even

that they enjoyed a lower cancer rate. These non-meat-eating women had a 40 percent lower mortality rate from uterine cancer and a 30 percent lower death rate from cancer of the breast. (Most of them, presumably, had once been meat eaters and this may have kept their cancer rate from being still lower.)

One isolated but interesting incident is reported by a nutritionally oriented physician from California, Henry Bieler. In his book *Food Is Your Best Medicine* Dr. Bieler briefly describes how he cured an actress's tumor by suppressing animal protein in her diet. In 1977 Gloria Swanson admitted that she was the actress. As Miss Swanson describes it, she came to Dr. Bieler in the 1940s with a tumor in her uterus. Three gynecologists had all decreed that a hysterectomy was required. But Miss Swanson did not, as she put it, want to give up being a woman at the age of forty-seven. So she went to Dr. Bieler to see if he could help.

Bieler pointed out that protein was a "cell-builder" and urged her to stay away from animal protein for at least a few years. Miss Swanson rigorously followed his advice. Two and a half years later she went back to consult one of the gynecologists she had originally seen. He somewhat reluctantly confirmed what she already felt to be the case, that the tumor had disappeared. However, when she told the specialist that she got rid of it by diet, he merely laughed. And when she added that it was a non-animal-protein diet that did it, he laughed all the louder.

A Dutch physician named Cornelius Moerman calls attention to his country's experience with cancer during World War II. The German occupiers of Holland expropriated nearly all the country's supplies of butter, meat, and cheese. The Dutch were left with few sources of nourishment other than grains, plus the vegetables they could grow in their own yards. As a result, says Dr. Moerman, the Dutch cancer rate during the German occupation dropped between 35 and 60 percent, depending on the type of malignancy involved.

People in Holland sometimes talk of the German food ex-
propriations as "the Adolf Hitler cancer cure."

If meat makes people more prone to malignant tumors,
then more than one factor in meat may bear the responsibil-
ity for doing so. The fat in meat tends to upset the hormonal
balance, as we have already learned from Dr. Berg's talk to
the National Cancer Institute. Some kinds of meat, as we
shall soon see, contain a carcinogen that we have encountered before. But the protein in meat may also prove to be a
potent provoker of cancer.

Some theories about protein, while they do not always
specifically point to any carcinogenic properties, leave the
possibility at least open. One, for which a certain amount of
evidence has accumulated, holds that protein molecules tend
to combine and, in turn, tend to clog the cells with debilitat-
ing and even dangerous debris. Another theory, developed
by some European researchers, holds that protein's absorption and utilization in the body produces a by-product called
amyloid. This by-product becomes deposited in the connective tissues, causing both tissues and organs to degenerate. A
third theory postulates that protein, through overstimulation
and irritation, encourages the abnormal cell growth that science associates with cancer.

At least one supernutritionist, Paavo Airola, Ph.D., has
expressed some concern about protein. Dr. Airola, who is
president of the International Academy of Biological
Medicine and a columnist for *Let's Live* magazine, says, "An
excess of animal protein can have a detrimental effect on
health, as well as may contribute to premature aging." A
nutrient that acts in this way seems likely to activate cancer.

Dr. Carlton Fredericks, president of the International
Academy of Preventive Medicine, raises another disturbing
point about protein. When a person's intake goes beyond
ninety grams a day, he says, the body starts to lose increased
amounts of calcium, phosphorous, iron, zinc, and magnesium. Since the last two minerals have been directly linked

with cancer deterrence, and since all of them are conducive to the good health that tends to curb cancer, high-protein diets may promote malignant tumor growth in still another way. Furthermore, other research shows that protein tends to remove vitamin A from our bodies as well. As a matter of fact, a British research team sent to drought-impacted Upper Volta in Africa in 1973 recommended that protein supplements *not* be sent to the undernourished people of the area. They feared it would create or accentuate vitamin A deficiencies.

All of these negative findings concerning protein should make all cancer-conscious Americans, as well as most other Western peoples, quite concerned. For high protein intake begins almost at birth for most of us. The modified cow's milk used as a substitute for breast milk by nonnursing mothers contains twice the amount of protein as human milk. Later, as an adult, the average American will consume nearly 100 grams of protein a day. Some of us actually absorb 130 to 140 grams a day.

Where does all this protein come from? Well, two large pork chops contain thirty-two protein grams. So does a quarter-pound hamburger on a roll. A corned beef sandwich has even more. It all adds up. As Dr. Ralph Nelson of the Mayo Medical School has pointed out, "Most people in this country eat perhaps twice as much protein as they need." In so doing, it might be added, we are eating more than is good for our health and well-being and, in the process, are probably making ourselves better prospects for becoming cancer patients.[1]

[1]An experiment conducted by a professor of medicine indicates that high-protein consumption can have other deleterious effects on the human body. Dr. Per-Olaf Astrand put nine male subjects on three different diets. For three days they ate a rather average diet consisting of proteins, fats, and carbohydrates. The next three days they consumed a diet high in protein and fats. And on the final three days they were given a carbohydrate-rich diet consisting largely of cereals, fruits, and vegetables.

We are now in a position to answer the question of what killed Adelle Davis. The double dose of radiation may have been the precipitating factor. But Miss Davis had doubtlessly developed some susceptibility to malignancy already, thanks to certain defects in her diet and life-style. These included a lack of vitamin C supplementation, the use of torula yeast as a substitute for brewer's yeast, the cigarettes, alcohol and drugs—along with the psychological stresses and strains that led to them—her indulgent view of fats, and her heavy intake of protein. Those of us who admire her dedication and agree with many of her ideas should learn still a further lesson from the misconceptions that may well have cost her her life.

Beef and the Bowel

Question: What other countries besides the United States suffer from a high incidence of cancer of the bowel and colon? Answer: Canada, New Zealand, Australia, and most of the nations of Western Europe, among others. Question: What do these nations have in common that makes this form of cancer so prevalent? Answer: A high rate of beef consumption.

Question: But shouldn't Argentina, then, have a high bowel cancer rate? After all, it is one of the leading beef-producing countries in the world. Answer: The bowel cancer

---

On the carbohydrate-rich diet, the men could pedal an average of 2 hours and 47 minutes on stationary bicycles before becoming fatigued. On the mixed diets, they averaged 1 hour and 57 minutes. And on the high-protein, high-fat diet, they lasted a mere 57 minutes on the average.

The June 1968 issue of *Nutrition Today*, in reporting the experiment, quoted Dr. Astrand as saying, "There seems no doubt that it is proper to exclude protein from consideration as a fuel for working muscle cells. . . . Forget the protein myth and the other superstitions."

rate of La Plata, Argentina, to take one example, is about *four times* the rate of that of Cali, Colombia, or Guatemala City, two other Latin American cities of similar cultures that consume much lower amounts of beef.

Indeed, the more one studies the statistics, the more amazed one becomes. Scotland, for example, has the highest bowel-colon cancer rate in the world with the worst incidence in and around Aberdeen, a famed center for cattle-raising. As a matter of fact, the Scottish death rate from this form of malignancy is 19 percent higher than the English. And as it happens, the Scots eat precisely 19 percent more beef than the English.

In the United States, the good people of Buffalo, New York, eat more beef per capita than the residents of Minneapolis–Saint Paul, who in turn consume more beef than the inhabitants of San Francisco, who, as it happens, ingest more beef than the citizens of Birmingham, Alabama. The death rates from bowel-colon cancer in these four cities adhere to precisely the same pattern. Buffalo has the highest, followed by Minneapolis–Saint Paul, San Francisco, and Birmingham, in that order. In general, the Southeast, which eats less beef and more pork and chicken, enjoys an appreciably lower bowel cancer death rate than does the rest of the country.

Finally, there are studies of various immigrant groups, such as the Japanese and the Poles. These studies show that such immigrants experience a bowel cancer rate that rises the longer and more completely they abandon the low-beef diets of their mother countries.

Dr. Berg of the National Cancer Institute, and his associate, Margaret Howell, Ph.D., presented these startling statistics to a national conference in 1973. In a subsequent article Dr. Howell wrote, "Beef or cattle meat is probably the most suspect of the meats. The evidence suggests that meat, particularly beef, is a food associated with the development of malignancies of the large bowel."

What are the possible reasons behind beef's apparent ability to produce bowel cancer? Dr. Berg, as we have already seen, believes that fat, especially animal fat, can create hormonal imbalances that can cause cancer. In addition, too much protein—especially, perhaps, meat protein—may also be a cancer producer. Since beef is pretty well packed with both fat and protein, it would already be a prime suspect. But in 1975 Dr. Raymond J. Shamberger of the Cleveland Clinic Foundation produced another piece of the puzzle. Beef, so he told the annual conference of the American Association for Cancer Research, contains an appreciable amount of malonaldehyde.

Now, we have come across malonaldehyde before. You may remember that unsaturated fats produce this substance when they become rancid. It is a powerful carcinogen. Dr. Shamberger and two of his colleagues once applied malonaldehyde to the shaved backs of mice. Within ten minutes these treated areas on the animals turned orange, and within three weeks over half of them had developed tumors. This experiment, together with some other studies, had prompted Shamberger and his two associates to conclude that "malonaldehyde might be the ultimate carcinogen."

Malonaldehyde, said Dr. Shamberger, is actually present in many foods. But, unlike beef, pork, chicken, and fish contain comparatively low levels of this noxious nutrient, while many fruits and vegetables contain none or almost none of it. However, nearly all foods tend to produce it when they decompose.

The lessons here are obvious. Don't leave leftover food lying around. Instead, wrap it well and place it in the refrigerator. Don't even keep it in the refrigerator longer than you have to. Those long-lived citizens of the southern Caucasus in the USSR, who do not have the refrigeration facilities that we enjoy, actually throw away their leftovers after every meal. Modern science has now shown how wise a practice this can be.

Dr. Shamberger also provides another useful tip. When you remove frozen meat from the freezer, allow extra time for it to thaw in the refrigerator with its wrapper still intact instead of trying to hurry up the process by thawing it at room temperature. Doing it the quicker way may only hasten the formation of malonaldehyde.

The most important lesson is the one we have already learned from examining the effects of fat and protein, only now we have another and still more persuasive reason for taking it to heart. Let us cut down on our consumption of meat, especially beef. Dr. Shamberger says that his research has caused him to reduce his meat consumption by nearly 50 percent. "Life is a series of risks," he observes. "As individuals and as a society we can and should identify the risks and reduce or eliminate as many as possible."

Sugar, Saccharin, and Salt

Dr. Gerson's diet, as we saw, called for rigidly suppressing all consumption of salt. He believed that sodium—salt is essentially a sodium compound—causes cancer. What evidence exists to prove him right?

For a long time no research findings were reported that showed any relationship between salt and cancer. All we had to go on were the successes Gerson had scored with his sodium-free diet. But in the January 1977 issue of *Let's Live*, Dr. Paavo Airola cited a study done on this subject in Japan by the World Health Organization. This research established a definite link between cancer and salt consumption.

Dr. Airola called attention to the study in connection with a trip that he made to Japan to lecture on nutrition and medicine. His own sojourn in the country uncovered ample evidence to confirm the study's conclusions. Of one of Japan's northern provinces known for its high rate of cancer he notes the following: "I found that their diet contains not only large amounts of salt, but also they eat very little fresh fruits and vegetables. Instead their diet contains lots of smoked fish, and practically all their vegetables are pickled with lots of salt."

The nutritional indictment against salt does not rest on its cancer-causing properties alone. As we already know, salt can contribute to, if not cause, high blood pressure, edema (water retention), and other health problems. Forcing the kidneys to eliminate large quantities of salt places these organs under substantial strain. In addition, salt seems to work at cross-purposes with potassium, a mineral that our bodies need and from which they derive great benefit, including, possibly, greater resistance to cancer. So we have plenty of reasons for reducing our consumption of salt.

Unfortunately, most of the foods that form the bulk of the modern diet contain copious quantities of salt, along with reduced reserves of potassium. For example, the U.S. Department of Agriculture informs us that 3½ ounces of fresh raw peas provide 316 milligrams of potassium and only 2 milligrams of sodium. But what happens when the peas become canned? A similar amount of canned peas on your supermarket shelf will contain 236 milligrams of sodium but only 96 milligrams of potassium. In other words, in the process of being canned, the peas undergo a hundred fold increase in sodium while losing more than two-thirds of their potassium.

Breakfast cereals offer another dismaying example of what happens when food becomes processed. The manufacturers of Wheaties, for example, boast that their product consists of whole wheat. And, so it does, which makes it probably one of the better of the standard breakfast cereals. However, a pound of whole wheat meal contains nearly

1,700 milligrams of potassium and only 9 milligrams of sodium, while a pound of Wheaties contains almost 4,700 milligrams of sodium and no potassium at all!

Salt is an inexpensive, but by no means an indispensable, way of improving food flavor. What we already know about the effect of too much salt, and of too little potassium, on our bodies should prompt us to keep our hands off the salt shaker as much as possible.

Sugar is another substance whose consumption has risen remarkably in recent years. The average American is now ingesting over two pounds of sugar and related sweeteners, such as corn syrup, every week. We know that sugar can cause or aggravate a variety of health problems. Can it cause cancer as well?

Probably no one knows as much about the harmful effects of sugar on the human body as Dr. John Yudkin. This British physician has spent most of his working lifetime studying sugar and has published several scientific reports, as well as one popularly oriented book, *Sweet and Dangerous.* Dr. Yudkin believes that sugar consumption may increase the likelihood that the consumer will contract certain forms of malignancy. However, he has devoted most of his time and attention to studying its more obvious ill effects on obesity, cholesterol, heart problems, and the like. In the meantime, several other findings, plus some of the well-known consequences of sugar, point to its possibilities as at least a catalyst for cancer.

The most well known, but apparently not highly feared, consequence of sugar is overweight. Some research indicates that overweight can create conditions that stimulate cancer. Dr. Roy L. Walford of the UCLA Medical School carried out some interesting experiments along these lines. He raised two groups of animals, one of which received their normal diet. The second group were given only one-third the calories of the first group, though all the vitamins, minerals, and other essential nutrients were supplied.

The result? The low-calorie animals not only lived 50 to 100 percent longer, but they developed 10 to 60 percent fewer tumors.

Such information as we have on humans shows similar patterns. One study shows that plump women tend to develop breast cancer somewhat more often than do slender women. Another study, involving 56,000 women who were members of TOPS (Take Off Pounds Sensibly), shows that women who were fat as teenagers and remain obese as adults run a 75 percent greater risk of developing cancer of the uterus lining than do women of normal weight.

It is also interesting to observe in this connection that in those three long-life and relatively cancer-free regions in the USSR, Pakistan, and Ecuador, caloric consumption falls far below the 2,400 calories a day that the U.S. Academy of Science recommends for males over fifty-five. The Hunzas consume a little over 1,900 calories a day. The estimated average for the south Russian group comes to 1,800 calories a day, while the Ecuadorian group thrive on about 1,200 calories a day.

One reason that sugar consumption increases our caloric intake is that sugar contains so little fiber. Indeed, it contains virtually no fiber at all. Hence, it fails to give us a feeling of satiation. We can go on eating it almost endlessly without feeling full.

This nearly total lack of roughage in sugar can aggravate another procancer condition. As we saw earlier, roughage tends to reduce the incidence of bowel and colon cancer. If high-fiber foods can protect us from intestinal cancer, then low-fiber foods, of which sugar is the supreme example, will most likely do the opposite.

Sugar, or at least refined white sugar, also tends to flush

certain valuable nutrients out of the body. These include magnesium, zinc, chromium as well as many, if not most, of the B vitamins. Since many of these food substances, as we have seen, appear to act against cancer, their loss leaves us less protected against the disease.

One very graphic and quite startling demonstration of sugar's deleterious effect on the human body was presented on the Merv Griffin show of April 25, 1977. Dr. Carlton Fredericks, who was appearing on the program, asked Griffin to hold one arm straight out while allowing the other arm to hang down at his side. Fredericks then proceeded to push the extended arm down while instructing Griffin to resist this pressure. As a result it took a good deal of effort to push the MC's extended arm down to the side. Fredericks then put a few lumps of sugar in the hand of Griffin's other arm, the one hanging down at his side. Fredericks again sought to push down the extended arm. This time, despite Griffin's efforts to resist, Dr. Fredericks easily brought it down.

Griffin raised the point that his arm's sudden weakness might not be due to the fact that the hand of his other arm was holding some sugar but that it was holding any object at all. However, when the experiment was repeated with Griffin holding some other object in the hand of his free arm, his extended arm stood up as well as when the hand of the other arm had been empty. It was only the presence of sugar in this hand that produced the surprising weakness in his arm.

The other guests on the show promptly proceeded to replicate the demonstration and, sure enough, when sugar cubes were held in the hand of the arm dangling at the side, the other arm, once extended, was easily pushed down. But when another object was placed in the free hand, or when it was left empty, the extended arm showed much more strength. After the show my wife and I tried the experiment ourselves and obtained the same results. Sugar held in the hand of one arm would immediately sap the strength of the other arm.

Another egregious effect of sugar is its effect on stress. As we saw in the previous chapter, stress can make us more cancer-prone, and strange as it may seem, sugar may actually increase stress. This at least is the view of Emanuel Cheraskin, M.D., a professor of medicine at the University of Alabama Medical Center and the author of thirteen books on nutrition. Dr. Cheraskin points out that sugar causes the pancreas to pump more insulin into the blood than the blood really needs. This excess insulin actually leads, within three hours, to a low blood sugar level. Low blood sugar levels make people irritable and, therefore, create stress. Dr. Carl Pfeiffer, the nutrition-oriented psychiatrist who directs the Brain-Bio Center in Princeton, New Jersey, agrees. Sugar, believe it or not, can stimulate stress.

Sugar can also apparently affect selenium, that "sleeper" trace mineral that tends to inhibit cancer. Two scientists with the U.S. Department of Agriculture report finding a striking decline in the selenium concentration in sugared breakfast cereals. In their opinion, the sugar dilutes the selenium.

Finally, and perhaps most importantly for our purposes, sugar directly and detrimentally affects our immunization system. One measurement used by doctors to judge the effectiveness of a person's immunication system is what is called the phagocytic index. This index is used in measuring the ability of the white cells to overcome toxic organisms in the blood. Two different research studies show that sugar serves to lower this highly crucial index. It thereby renders us more open to disease, including, it would seem, cancer.

One final fact is worth noting. The centenarians who inhabit the three long-life regions of the world eat very little or no sugar. However, those who live in the Soviet and Pakistani regions—I have no information on this point regarding the third region in Ecuador—do consume appreciable amounts of honey. This is further evidence that honey, for reasons that science has yet to learn, tends in some way to foster health and build protection from cancer.

Saccharin first appeared on the scene in the 1890s. However, it is only in recent decades that its use has become widespread. Its growing popularity has understandably triggered a good deal of research into its possible ill effects.

The first sign that it might produce cancer came in 1970 when researchers at the University of Wisconsin Medical School implanted saccharin pellets into the bladders of mice. They found that up to 52 percent of the mice developed bladder cancer.

In 1974, the Canadian government sponsored a study of its own to determine whether saccharin could be carcinogenic. The experiment involved feeding 100 rats a diet consisting of 5 percent pure saccharin from *conception* to death. (The saccharin feeding actually started with the rats' mothers while they were gestating.) Of the 100 saccharin-saturated rats, 14 had developed cancerous bladders by the time they died. In a control group of 100 rats who received no saccharin, only two of the animals developed such tumors.

The results prompted the Food and Drug Administration to ban the use of saccharin in all prepared foods, such as diet drinks. The sugar industry, which had itself sponsored much research into saccharin with the hope of proving it harmful, reacted jubilantly to the news. And the shares of sugar company stocks immediately rose on the New York Stock Exchange.

Others, however, did not find the news so sweet. They pointed out that a human being would have to consume some 800 bottles of diet soft drinks a day from birth to death in order to duplicate the amount of the artificial sweetener given the test animals. Furthermore, even after such massive and continuous dosages, only 12 percent more rats developed bladder tumors than those who received no saccharin.

As the controversy continued, other studies came to light indicating that saccharin presented few, if any, dangers to human beings. Alexander Marble, M.D., the director of the Joslin Diabetes Foundation, cited two of them as he sought to rebut the FDA's claim.

One was conducted by Dr. Joseph Kessler in 1970. Dr. Kessler examined the medical records of more than 21,000 diabetes patients seen at the Joslin Clinic over a twenty-six year period. He found that their rate of bladder cancer roughly paralleled that of the general population. Since diabetics consume, on the average, much more saccharin than the general population, one would expect to find a higher cancer rate among them if saccharin posed any dangers.

The other study cited by Dr. Marble dealt with a group of rhesus monkeys who were given heavy doses of saccharin over a six-year period. None of these developed bladder cancer.

All in all, the total evidence suggests that the peril that saccharin presents to the normal human consumer is indeed slight, if not actually nonexistent. Furthermore, even such slight danger as it may present can be further minimized by taking two precautionary steps. The first is to take a vacation from saccharin for a few days every now and then. This suggestion comes from Carlton Fredericks, who points out that while small amounts of the sweetener may accumulate in the kidney over a period of regular usage, research indicates that the saccharin quickly dissolves and disappears when consumption ceases. The second step is even simpler. It consists of simply taking a goodly amount of vitamin C. This vitamin, as we have seen, has already proven itself to be a powerful inhibitor of bladder cancer.

Cigarettes, Caffeine, and Alcohol

Lung cancer kills more Americans than any other form of cancer and nine out of ten of its victims smoke or have smoked cigarettes. These facts fortunately, are well known. Less well known is the fact that cigarette smoking may also play a role in other forms of cancer as well. Dr. Meera Jain of the University of Toronto's Department of Preventive Medicine has found a correlation between cigarette smoking and bladder cancer. The National Cancer Institute and other researchers have reported similar findings. One urologist says he has never seen a bladder cancer patient who didn't smoke.

But if smoking can cause bladder cancer, so also can alcohol. Dr. Jain claims to have found such a correlation, and so has the National Cancer Institute. In September 1974 the institute reported some research from UCLA demonstrating that bladder cancer death rates were highest in states that had the highest beer consumption.

The possible carcinogenic effects of alcohol are not limited to the bladder. The Third National Cancer Survey found a positive association between alcohol and breast, thyroid, and skin cancers. This discovery prompted Dr. Roger R. Williams, a professor of medicine at the University of Utah, to do a more detailed study. He found that drinking increased the chances of breast cancer in women 20 to 60 percent, of thyroid cancer in men and women 30 to 150 percent, and of skin cancer in both sexes 20 to 70 percent. What's more, even people who consumed as little as one drink a month ran at least a slightly greater risk of contracting cancer than did teetotalers.

Of course, statistical correlations can be tricky. Many people who drink also smoke cigarettes. And it is possible that drinkers, even light drinkers, may as a group suffer from greater stress and eat less nutritionally than nondrinkers. But Dr. Williams believes that there is a distinct and direct cause-and-effect relationship. Alcohol, he says, "stimulates the secretion of hormones in the pituitary gland which speeds up cell reproduction—and this increases susceptibility to the development of a malignancy." Dr. James Eustrom of UCLA, who has also done some research in this area, concurs. In his view, alcohol may increase cell production and thereby produce cancer.

The investigations that have been done into the relationship between smoking and cancer and between alcohol and cancer are certainly impressive. The data these researchers have compiled are both massive and persuasive. The theories they advance strike medical experts and laymen as quite convincing. But they run into one problem. In some of the long-life regions of the world, drinking and cigarette smoking are quite common.

In the Soviet group, wine is consumed at both lunch and dinner, and a certain amount of vodka is imbibed as well. Some of these healthy centenarians smoke cigarettes, a few of them quite heavily. In the Ecuadorian group, the predisposition to indulgence in such vices seems even greater. Dr. David Davies, a British scientist who visited them, found that many of them smoke forty to sixty cigarettes a day and drink up to four cups of rum daily. How do we explain their long life and relative freedom from cancer in the face of such "perverse" behavior?

As for smoking, one explanation may lie in the question of inhalation. To put it more simply, they may simply not inhale the smoke. We know that pipe and cigar smokers have nowhere near the lung cancer rate of those who smoke cigarettes. They do, to be sure, have higher rates for lip and tongue cancer, but these are still fairly rare and, more importantly, they are rarely fatal. The annals of history show numerous personages who lived well into their eighties and even nineties while puffing away on cigars and pipes. The list includes such distinguished and diverse figures as Winston Churchill, Bertrand Russell, General Douglas MacArthur, Herbert Hoover, Pablo Casals, George Meany, and former House Speaker John MacCormack. (The last two gentlemen, at this writing, are still very much alive.)

Another possible, and not incompatible, reason that the centenarians of the USSR and Ecuador are able to smoke cigarettes with comparative immunity may lie in the nature of the tobacco they use. Both groups grow their own tobacco, and it may be that their tobacco leaves contain far fewer carcinogenic components than ours.

As it happens, evidence has arisen in recent years indicating that differences in the tobacco itself can create differences in the degrees of danger that smokers encounter. One writer, William Dufty, advances the novel argument that it is the sugar content of the tobacco that is responsible. In his book *Sugar Blues,* Dufty claims that in the Soviet Union, Japan, and Formosa, cigarette smoking does not show any marked correlation with lung cancer. The tobacco used in these countries, he says, is cured in such a way as to leave it without any appreciable amount of sugar. Western countries, however, use a different curing process, one that gives their tobacco a relatively high sugar content.

To buttress his point further, Dufty notes that English tobacco contains somewhat more sugar than American tobacco, which in turn harbors more sugar than the tobacco smoked in France. Sure enough, England's lung cancer rate exceeds ours, and ours tops that of France.

Dufty's thesis is intriguing and even impressive. Of course, other factors may also be at work. In England, for instance, the comparatively high price of cigarettes causes many smokers to smoke their butts down to the very end. This alone could account for the country's greater rate of lung cancer. Nevertheless, differences of one kind or another in the tobacco itself may be one reason that some of the Russian and Ecuadorian long-lived individuals can apparently smoke, and possibly even inhale, cigarettes with relative impunity.

The drinking they do poses a greater dilemma. However, we do know that the vodka that the South Russian group drinks comes, like their wine, from grapes. Now grapes are a quite wholesome food. They contain some vitamins, including vitamin E, and some minerals. They are especially rich in potassium, the mineral that Dr. Gerson made the cornerstone of his diet. Like all fruits, they are very low in protein. Though they contain sugar, the sugar is interwoven with other natural substances and is not likely to do the damage that white refined sugar does. In the Soviet Union generally, grapes are considered a medicinal food, and grape diets are sometimes prescribed by Soviet physicians for certain types of illness.

Explaining the rum consumed by the Ecuadorian old-agers poses greater problems. It may contain some substances that render it less harmful. Those who consume it may have special constitutions that enable them to resist any of its ill effects. Or the other positive elements in their diets and life-styles may make them immune from its evils.

The conclusion we can draw from all this would seem to be that while we will be better off not smoking or drinking at all, we can probably smoke even American tobacco without inhaling and sip a bit of wine without great danger. Certainly millions upon millions have done so and have managed to lead long and cancer-free lives.

But what about another and even more commonly used produce—coffee? Can it cause cancer?

There are those who think it can. In 1971 Dr. Philip Cole of the Harvard School of Public Health reported "an unanticipated finding" linking coffee consumption with bladder cancer. He expressed the opinion that one-fourth of all such cases in men and one-half of all such cases in women came from coffee drinking. Those women who drank even a cup a day appeared to run two and a half times more risk of developing bladder cancer than did non–coffee drinkers.

Two years later, two researchers at Rosewell Park Memorial Institute in Buffalo reported finding that most bladder cancer patients were regular coffee drinkers. Very few reported that they drank little or no coffee.

We do know that caffeine is a drug that can damage the human body. Among other things, it can deplete the body of certain B vitamins. Even the somewhat lesser amounts found in tea may have this effect. A University of Hawaii study, for example, found that volunteer test subjects who dránk four to six cups of tea a day demonstrated vitamin B deficiencies despite the fact that they consumed a nutritionally adequate diet.

Such studies suggest that we should take care to keep our coffee and tea drinking within moderation. They also underline the importance of taking vitamins. These include not just the B vitamins, but also vitamin C, whose effectiveness in combating bladder cancer we have already seen.

Getting It While It's *Not* Hot

In traditional Chinese families the men fairly frequently develop mouth cancer. The women rarely do. Does this attest to the greater powers of the Chinese female to resist cancer? Not necessarily. A researcher who looked into the question came up with a different answer. He found that in the Chinese family the man, being firmly ensconced as head of the house, is always served the soup first. Consequently, he starts to consume it when it is still steaming. Hence his greater susceptibility to cancer of the mouth.

Eating foods that are too hot can cause other forms of cancer as well. Some research done at the University of Tokyo found that continuous consumption of scalding hot beverages and hot foods can lead to cancer of the throat, esophagus, and stomach, as well as cancer of the mouth. And Dr. Airola in his study of the cancer-prone province in northern Japan mentioned earlier found that its inhabitants "eat their rice extremely hot and also drink scalding hot teas and soups."

Many have long suspected that eating hot foods could produce cancer. We now see that their suspicions were well founded.

How Improving Your Looks Can Give You Cancer

An anticancer diet and life-style will generally tend to improve one's appearance. For that fringe benefit we can all be grateful. But some practices that many women and some men undertake to make themselves look better may expose them to considerable risk of cancer. Indeed, one practice pursued with the aim not only of looking more attractive but also of looking healthier may actually achieve the opposite effect. This is the practice of sunbathing.

The sun, which is the primary source of so much energy, is also the primary source of skin cancer. Those who needlessly expose themselves to its ultraviolet rays may be setting themselves up for trouble. Ironically enough, they will also, over a period of time, make themselves less attractive, since the sun causes wrinkles. "I think sunlight ages the skin more than anything else," says Dr. Alexander Fisher, Clinical Professor of Dermatology at New York University's Post Graduate Medical School. He adds, "Most people don't realize that the sunburn they had twenty years ago can cause skin cancer and wrinkles today."

Many people who are aware of the cause-and-effect relationship between sunlight and skin cancer shrug off the warning it implies by noting that skin cancer is rarely fatal. To be sure, less than 2 percent of those who contract this malignancy die as a result. But that less-than-2-percent figure, nevertheless, translates into over 5,000 deaths a year. That just about equals the combined number of people who die from cancer of the bone, cancer of the thyroid, and cancer of the connective tissue. Victorian women who believed that a pale, even pallid, face was a sign of beauty, may have known something which we are just beginning to realize.

Some recently revealed research points a strong finger of suspicion at another, and more artificial, beauty aid as a cause of cancer in women. This is hair dye. Bruce N. Ames, Ph.D., of the National Academy of Sciences has examined 169 hair dyes. Using a test he has developed, Dr. Ames found that 150 of them contain materials that he has found to be often carcinogenic. At the National Cancer Institute, Dr. Elizabeth Weisburger has fed hair dye ingredients to rats, only to see some of the animals develop unanticipated tumors.

But hair dyes, you may respond, are applied only externally. Many other chemical compounds, such as alcohol, would also be dangerous if ingested but may be used on the skin with relative safety. Why not hair dyes as well?

The answer is that some of the substances found in such coloring agents have turned up in the urine of some of the women using them. And at least one physician, Dr. Nathan Shafer of New York City, claims to have spotted a strong coincidence between women who dye their hair and those who develop breast cancer. He says that 87 percent of his nearly 100 breast cancer patients are long-term users of hair coloring. This compares to only 30 percent of the general female population in the relevant age-group who dye their hair.

Obviously more study needs to be done on this subject before definitive conclusions can be drawn. But the evidence already in is sufficient to post a warning signal.

Does a Technological Society Create Cancer?

The technological society has brought us many wonders. But in the minds of many, these include a rising rate of cancer. Its new devices and delights, its practices and processes, have left a growing incidence of malignancy in their wake.

Take the subject of chemicals. Modern society makes increasing use of these compounds. Yet, Dr. Umberto Saffiotti of the National Cancer Institute says some 1,000 of them have been found to be carcinogenic. Dr. Leo Friedman, a toxicologist with the Food and Drug Administration, seems to go even farther. Chemicals, he claims, are responsible for nine out of every ten cancer cases in the country.

One aspect of this problem is pollution. Studies have shown, or at least indicated, that people who live by a busy highway are more likely to contract cancer than those who reside several streets back. New Jersey, which is our most industrialized state, also happens to be the state with the highest incidence of cancer.

Some of these pollutants plague us by getting into our water supply. Dr. Berg of the National Cancer Institute reported in 1972 that he had found many cancer-causing substances in various water systems. Those areas served by a water system containing appreciable amounts of lead tended to have increased incidence of stomach, intestinal, ovarian, kidney, and blood cancer. Where beryllium was present, bone, breast, and uterine cancer seemed to be high. Arsenic and nickel also correlated with certain forms of cancer, while the substance that correlated most closely with fatal malignancy overall was cadmium.

Our food supply is also believed to have become endangered. Many of the commonly used fertilizers are suspected. Some of these fertilizers seem to have increased the fluorine content of food. In 1965 researchers at the University of Texas found that adding fluorine to the drinking water of mice caused tumors that had been transplanted into the animals to grow at a faster rate. Sweden, as a matter of fact, has now banned the use of fluoridation in its water supplies, ruling it to be an unsafe additive. (However, the National Cancer Institute sees no danger in fluorine.)

The possible effect of chemicals on our food supply remains, as yet, quite controversial. There certainly is much evidence on both sides. But one report should make us all start to wonder. A Dr. Donald C. Collins has claimed to know of five cancer patients who cured themselves *simply by eating organically grown food.* "The only constant factor in the lives of these five persons," said Dr. Collins, "was the fact that they all ate home-raised organically grown foods that were free from chemical preservatives and insect repellant sprays." However, Dr. Vachon wisely cautions anyone not to rely on such an approach alone as a means of curing himself or herself of cancer.

Even some of the medical wonders designed to help our health seem to have helped the cancer rate to grow. From 1969 to 1973, a period of only four years, the incidence of uterine cancer in the country shot up dramatically, as much as 60 percent in some areas. During the same time, the dollar value of estrogen prescriptions given to women to assist them with menopausal problems more than doubled. Some began wondering if some relationship did not exist between these two events. Sure enough, research now shows that women who take estrogen run an eight times greater risk of incurring cancer than those in their age group who forego this medical "aid." (Carlton Fredericks, by the way, warned physicians about this danger when they first began giving estrogen injections in the 1950s. Unfortunately, his advice went unheeded.)

Then, there is the matter of diethylstibestrol, or, as it is more commonly known, DES. Some years ago doctors began giving this drug to women for a variety of conditions. Evidence now shows that its ill effects can be, and have been, transmitted to the recipients' offspring. Vaginal cancer in several hundred young women and teenage girls has been traced to the DES administered to their mothers during pregnancy.

Dr. Roger R. Williams, whose studies of the effect of alcohol on cancer were cited a few pages earlier, says his studies indicate that many drugs commonly prescribed by doctors cause cancer. At the head of the list he places reserpine, a medicine commonly used to curb high blood pressure. He blames this drug alone for possibly causing 5,000 cancer cases a year. Other drugs he suspects include methyldopa, phenothiazine, d-amphetamine, and some antidepressants and other antihistamines.

Other danger may come from the X ray machines that physicians and hospitals have made increasing use of in recent years, not only for diagnosis, but for treating tonsillitis and even acne. The International Commission on Radiological Protection has indicated that current X ray usage in the United States is producing 3,000 deaths a year from various forms of cancer and genetic damage. What's more, such present use of X rays may cause ten times as many future deaths from cancer and other problems. One of the country's foremost experts on radiation, Dr. John W. Gofman of the University of California at Berkeley, notes that "all responsible authorities agree there is *no* evidence for any 'safe' threshold dose of radiation."

One conclusion from all this is inescapable: many doctors using the most modern means of medicine, have only succeeded in causing more cancer than they have cured.

But having taken the technological society, including some of its medicine, to task, we should now pause to examine its more positive points. Such positive points do exist, though many critics often lose sight of them.

To begin with, the society that preceded it was no bed of roses in terms of health or most anything else. If the cancer rate has risen relentlessly in recent years, this could stem from the fact that science has snuffed out or suppressed so many other diseases. In other words, many, perhaps most, of the people now falling victim to cancer would have succumbed to other diseases earlier in their lives if they had lived in former times. The growing incidence of cancer may simply reflect the fact that people with weaker immunization systems are now living long enough to contract it. This in no way softens the peril that cancer poses, but it does help us put it in perspective.

Many of the cancer-causing conditions that exist today did not exist, say, at the turn of the century. But other conditions that can cause cancer or other forms of disease were worse. Cities without cars did not have to contend with pollution exhaust, but think of what the air must have been like with all those coal and wood-burning stoves and furnaces going. Think of the gallons of urine and tons of manure that the horses dumped on the streets of American cities every day.

Our food, to be sure, grew to ripening without the aid of chemicals. But think of the worms, molds, and other infestations that could contaminate it. And think of the putrefaction that must often have set in before refrigeration. (Think of all the cancer-causing malonaldehyde, for one thing, that this must have spawned.)

Furthermore, the correlations between pollution and cancer do not always hold up. If New Jersey has the highest cancer rate, then rural Maine and New Hampshire are not far behind. Parts of those states have among the highest cancer death rates in the country. When it comes to cities, Baltimore enjoys the dubious distinction of having the highest cancer rate for white males. Baltimore has a fair number of factories, but it is less industralized than Gary, Indiana, Pittsburgh, Pennsylvania, and many other cities. Furthermore, from 1955 to 1975 the air in most American cities became distinctly cleaner, but the cancer rate failed to respond by going down or even leveling off.

Looking around the world, we find many similar situations. Brittany and Normandy are two of France's most rural provinces, but they are not among those provinces with the lowest rate of cancer. Japan is the most heavily industrialized, and far and away the most heavily polluted, nation in the world. Up until recently, Japanese traffic policemen sometimes had to wear masks to keep from succumbing to noxious fumes. Yet, Japan ranks quite low in all of the most fatal forms of malignancy except stomach cancer. And its high rate of stomach cancer is blamed not on its industrialized environment but on the dietary habits of its citizens. As we saw earlier, they tend to consume many highly salted and smoked foods.

We should also bear in mind that while natural foods can help deter cancer, a few of them may actually bring it on. For example, cancer of the esophagus is unusually high in the pleasant Caribbean island of Curaçao. Researchers believe that carcinogens found in plant extracts on the island are responsible. And although Africa has much less cancer than the Western world, some African tribes do show high rates for certain types of cancer, and again researchers blame carcinogens in certain foods that they consume. (Beetlenut is sometimes identified as a cancer-causing plant.) This shows that nature does not provide blanket protection from cancer. It, too, on occasion, may prove harmful.

Finally, a few of the chemicals used to protect our food supply may actually help protect us from cancer. The antioxidants known as BHT and BHA come especially to mind. Although some nutritionists frown upon them, Dr. Denham Harman of the University of Nebraska Medical School found that mice fed regular amounts of these chemicals over a long period of time lived nearly 50 percent longer than they customarily do. Furthermore, one form of malignancy, stomach cancer, has actually declined quite precipitously since the 1930s, and some observers believe that the introduction of these preservatives into breakfast cereals and other foods may have caused this welcome development.

None of this is meant to give the current use of chemicals a clean bill of health. Certainly not. Nor should we relax our vigil regarding any of the other aspects of contemporary life that may be cancer-conducive. However, it does mean that the cancer challenge we confront can be met as long as we take reasonable environmental precautions and as long as we keep our personal immunization systems in good working order.

Living
the Anticancer Life

Living the anticancer life may be easier than you think. It does not, for most people, necessitate any dramatic changes in life-style. If, for example, you enjoy city life, you should not immediately pack up your bags and head for the hills to escape the effects of pollution. (There's cancer in the hills, too, as the cancer death rates of Maine, New Hampshire, and many other rural states grimly attest.) Furthermore, those changes that an anticancer regimen does call for yield tangible and immediate joys and rewards of their own.

The most stressful and most obvious change that is called for is the one that confronts cigarette smokers. They should, especially if they are males, give them up. Transcendental meditation can be of real use here. Many have found it comparatively easy to break the habit after meditating only a week or two. The B vitamins can also help. Taken in heavy amounts, they tend to soothe the nerves.

While it is better to smoke nothing at all, many, although

not all, of the ill effects of tobacco can be avoided by simply smoking without inhaling. If you do smoke cigarettes and find it impossible to give up tobacco completely, then you should consider switching to cigars or pipes. This, too, requires a readjustment and, in the case of pipes, some knowledge of how to smoke them. But the readjustment is a lot easier than that required for giving up smoking completely. Once it is made, most people who have made it find that they would never return to cigarettes, even if cigarettes became harmless.

The advice on switching to cigars or pipes as a substitute for giving up smoking completely is not addressed to men alone. There are many pipes and small cigars on the market these days for women, and many women now smoke them. To repeat, it is certainly better to smoke nothing at all, but it is far better to smokes pipes or cigars than to continue inhaling cigarettes.

If you find that you simply cannot give up cigarettes, then at least choose brands low in tar and nicotine, leave long butts, and fortify yourself as much as possible against their ill effects. Among other things, you should take extra amounts of vitamin A, C, and E (we will be discussing these vitamins shortly).

By all means try to reduce the amount of stress in your life. Cut down on the changes and choices that you make, and when you do have to make a major change, try to keep the other elements of your life stable. You should also make sure that you have ways and means of expressing your feelings. If this is difficult for you, then you should consider discussing the problem with a clergyman or counselor. Suppressing your sentiments and emotions sets you up for possible malignancy.

By all means keep yourself physically active. If you are middle-aged or older, you should especially give some thought to walking regularly. Unless you have a heart problem and your doctor has told you not to, walk hills and stairs as well. It is probably no coincidence that the three long-living regions of the world that we have examined are all located in hilly country, forcing their residents to spend a good deal of time and effort going up and down slopes.

In this country there is no region known for its number of long-living and cancer-free people, but there is a town that once attracted the attention of many observers because of its low heart attack rate. This is Roseta, Pennsylvania, a small community made up mostly of Italian-Americans. Roseta long boasted the lowest heart attack rate in the United States, despite the fact that its citizens consumed generous amounts of heavy, cholesterol-laden foods. Some of the reason for their low susceptibility may lie in the fact that they ate sizable amounts of garlic and some other healthful and heart-protecting foods. But another factor may be that Roseta lies along the side of a hill, and its residents find themselves having to go up and down it constantly.

Be sure, of course, when you are out walking or doing anything else outdoors to protect yourself from too much sun. Those ultraviolet rays can prove lethal, especially for fair-complexioned people. Sunshine is healthy, but only up to a point.

Take annual, or even semiannual, checkups if you wish, but do not count upon them. You can walk out of your doctor's office with a clean bill of health only to start developing cancer symptoms in a week or two. Count instead upon following doctors' rules and observing those practices to which scientific evidence points as being cancer-protective.

Food Supplements

Food supplements probably play the cardinal role in cancer-deterrence. For one thing, they enable us to reap the benefits that accrue from taking helpful substances in more

concentrated and more copious amounts. By making extensive use of such supplements, we can also avoid making
sweeping and often physically impossible changes in our
daily diets.

The most important of these food substances, and probably the most important overall component of an anticancer
regimen, is vitamin C. Take at least 2,000 milligrams of this
valuable vitamin every day. Vitamins seem to work best when
food is present in the stomach for them to work on, so take
your vitamin C right after breakfast. In this way you know
that whatever happens to you that day, you will have obtained your daily ration of this useful vitamin and at a time
when your system is best geared to make use of it.

This doesn't mean that you should not take vitamin C at
other times of the day. On the contrary, if you took 500
milligrams four times a day after meals or snacks, it would
probably benefit you even more. But taking 2,000 milligrams
right after breakfast guarantees that you will have your daily
ration. Therefore, it is probably the best practice for most of
us to follow. Additional amounts of vitamin C can be consumed later on if you so desire.

Other vitamins, as we have learned, are also important.
How much of them should you take? It depends, somewhat,
on the state of your health, your age, and other factors. Un-
healthy people need more vitamins than healthy ones, and
older people, since their bodies do not use vitamins as effectively, need more than younger people. Vitamin A can be
taken in daily amounts ranging up to 25,000 units; vitamin E,
in amounts ranging up to 2,500 units. As for the B vitamins,
they can be consumed in almost unlimited amounts.

But isn't there some danger, you may wonder, in taking
too much? The danger of vitamin overdosage is very slight,
and such amounts as I have mentioned would scarcely be
enough to create any peril. Vitamin A and vitamin D are
considered to present the greatest danger, and that is why

the Food and Drug Administration has decreed that no vitamin pill can contain more than 10,000 units of vitamin A. Cases of vitamin A overdosages are very rare, however, with most of them occurring in children. There are over 50,000 units of vitamin A in a four-ounce serving of beef-liver and over 15,000 units in a normal serving of carrots. Eskimos eating their normal diet consume 200,000 to 300,000 units of vitamin A a day. (Most Eskimos no longer eat their regular diet, thanks to the increasing inroads made by civilization. As a result, they now experience far more health problems.)

To put your mind further to rest on this point, consider the following. The Nobel prize–winning physician Whipple put his patients on a diet of eating raw liver three times a day. (He received his Nobel prize for his discovery that liver stopped the progress of pernicious anemia.) Under this diet, the patients received about 250,000 units of vitamin A a day over a long period of time. Whipple never reported noticing any signs of hypervitaminosis, as vitamin overdosage is called. Another Nobel prize winner in chemistry, Linus Pauling, has pointed out that there is "very little danger of damage through hypervitaminosis A. . . ." It should be noted that in those rare cases where such hypervitaminosis does occur, it is easily corrected by simply reducing the dosage.

What about vitamin C? Being what is called a water-soluble vitamin, as are the B vitamins, it washes out of the body easily. However, some evidence has arisen to suggest that in heavy doses it can be somewhat threatening. In late 1974 the *Journal of the American Medical Association* carried a report stating that vitamin C tended to destroy vitamin B_{12} and therefore could cause anemia. However, soon other evidence appeared that indicated the extreme unlikelihood of this ever happening. A group of hospitals in Saint Louis, for example, had been giving 4,000 milligrams of vitamin C a day to all their spinal cord injury patients. They promptly tested these patients when they read the *Journal*'s report, but found none of them to be deficient in vitamin B_{12}, though each had been receiving the heavy dose of vitamin C for more than eleven months.

Another report in 1975 told of finding that massive doses of vitamin C given to laboratory animals on an empty stomach produced genetic damage in some of the animals. But the amounts given, adjusted for the greater body weight of humans, would involve much more vitamin C than we are talking about. If Dr. Charles Butterworth, the former chairman of the American Medical Association's Food and Nutrition Council, believes that 2,000 milligrams a day of vitamin C is safe, then we should have no qualms about consuming such an amount. (I personally take nearly 4,000 units a day and greatly increase this amount whenever I feel a cold coming on. Vitamin C greatly reduces the incidence of colds in most people but doesn't end them altogether.)

Vitamin E has also been found to be harmless in fairly large doses. Two researchers at the National Institutes of Health tested twenty-eight adults who were taking up to 800 units of this vitamin a day. After extensive tests, the researchers concluded that "no signs of toxicity were uncovered in this investigation." As a matter of fact, most of the subjects studied said they had noticed specific improvements in their health since taking the vitamin.

Dr. Evan Shute, the Canadian cardiologist probably knows more about vitamin E than anyone else, since he and his brother, who is also a physician, have used it on 30,000 patients. Dr. Shute offers some interesting material on this point. He suggests a dosage of 400 units a day for an average normal woman and 600 units a day for an average normal man. He himself takes 2,400 units a day because he feels that his advancing years make him "vulnerable." (He does recommend, however, that persons with high blood pressure work into vitamin E slowly, starting by taking only 100 units a day and then gradually increasing the amount.)

The B vitamins have also been found to be innocuous in relatively large doses. In one test, for example, volunteers were given 10,000 milligrams of pantothenic acid daily for six weeks, and no harmful effects were observed. Of course, virtually any food substance can do you damage if you take enormous quantities of it over a long period of time. It is thought by many nutritionists that you need have no fears about taking several hundred milligrams of the B vitamins every day; others disagree.

A further question that confronts us concerns the relative advantages of what are called natural vitamins versus synthetic ones. Even the experts that we tend to rely on break ranks on this. Linus Pauling and Roger A. Williams, both chemists, generally feel that the synthetics offer the same values as those derived from natural sources. Whether a vitamin is taken from a food or concocted in a laboratory, they emphasize, its chemistry remains the same. Consequently, we should take advantage of the lower costs entailing in producing vitamins synthetically.

Others, however, disagree. Dr. Samuel Ayers, Jr., a Los Angeles physician, claims a difference does exist. Writing in the *Journal of the American Medical Association*, he points out that this presumed sameness between synthetic and natural vitamins is certainly not true of vitamin E. While the natural and synthetic forms appear chemically identical, "they affect polarized light differently and in animal experiments the *d* or natural form is considerably more active than the *dl* or synthetic form." He quoted several research studies to back up his claim. One showed the natural form of vitamin as having a 20 percent greater potency than the synthetic form.

Vitamin C in a natural form comes mixed with certain substances known as the bioflavonoids. While the Food and Drug Administration maintains that these accompanying substances have no known nutritional value, others strongly dispute this. Among these dissenters is Dr. Albert Szent-

Gyorgyi, the research physician who won the Nobel prize for discovering vitamin C. Dr. Szent-Gyorgyi claims that the bioflavonoids improve the action of the capillaries and, among other things, can help prevent or alleviate hemorrhoids. Dr. Emanuel Cheraskin and Dr. Carlton Fredericks also believe that the bioflavonoids are useful nutrients.

Turning to vitamin A, we find that the natural form derived from fish oils gives you actually a complex of vitamins. The cluster of compounds is not only believed by some, at least, to be more effective, but it also has been judged to be less toxic. Among those rare cases of overdosage of this vitamin, there are no cases where such overdose occurred as the result of taking the vitamin in its natural form.

Viewing the whole question of natural versus synthetic vitamins, Dr. Isabel Jennings writes, in her book *Vitamins in Endocrine Metabolism*, "In many ways synthetic vitamins are now available which may be identical with the naturally occurring substance or only closely related. The close relations, although useful in many ways, pose some problems in that they may have only a fraction, whether large or small, of the biological activity of the natural product. They may substitute for several, but not all, of the functions of their natural counterparts, so that it is essential to use extreme care in their use."

Another scientist shares this view. Writing in his book *Clinical Physiology*, Dr. Jonathan Forman says, "It is a great mistake to assume that a synthetic imitation is *biologically* identical to the natural counterpart. There are many ways in which they may be chemically alike but where the natural product is quite different *biologically*. The chemist has no such methods as the living cell for distinguishing subtle differences." (Emphasis added.)

Still another scientist takes an even more negative view. Joseph M. Kadans, Ph.D., says many nonnatural vitamins are derived from synthesizing coal or wood tar and therefore "may actually be toxic."

Thus, you are probably better off taking natural vitamins. If the expense seems prohibitive, then take some of each. For example, I take 2,500 to 3,000 milligrams of vitamin C after breakfast. This is usually simple ascorbic acid, synthetically made. However, during the course of the day, I usually munch on a few 100-milligram tablets of natural vitamin C to make sure I am obtaining the bioflavonoids and any other benefits that the natural form may have to bestow.

Many minerals are also available in supplement form. These include magnesium and zinc, both of which I take religiously (30 or more milligrams of zinc and up to 300 milligrams of magnesium). Brewer's yeast and desiccated liver are also obtainable in tablet form and may be consumed for their minerals (such as selenium), their nucleic acid, their vitamins, and any other valuable nutrients they may have. Even pollen and yogurt are available as tablets.

It is important to take a balance of supplements. For example, too much vitamin E or C can reduce the amount of vitamin A stored in your body, so for this reason alone, you should not take them without some vitamin A as well. The B vitamins, as we have seen, tend to interact with one another, and too much of one can cause a deficiency in another, if you are not careful to take them all. Magnesium must be present in the body for vitamin C and possibly the B vitamins to work effectively. But magnesium itself will increase the need for calcium. (Dolomite, a compound sold in health food stores, contains a suitable balance of calcium and magnesium and therefore provides a good method for safely increasing one's magnesium intake. The calcium, by the way, while it has no known effect on cancer, is valuable for your overall health in many ways.) Finally, vitamin E seems to work most effectively when a fair amount of selenium is present and vice versa.

A few of these supplements, such as brewer's yeast or magnesium, tend to give some people gas. If this happens to you, then mix two teaspoons of apple cider vinegar into the water you use to wash them down, and, if necessary, take another glass or two of the same mixture later in the day. As we grow older, the amount of hydrochloric acid in our stomachs tend to decline, hence our increasing disposition to generate gas. Apple cider vinegar, besides providing other health benefits, helps alleviate this problem.

You may become aghast at all the pills you have to take, and you may feel that you cannot or should not swallow so many. However, you should remember that these tablets are not drugs but simply concentrated forms of food. Twelve brewer's yeast tablets seem like a lot, but they represent only a tablespoon of the food itself. Hence to get the full value of such food supplementation, you should not balk at taking too many tablets. They not only will provide you with some valuable protection against cancer but will contribute greatly to your overall health and happiness.

Diet

Although food supplements offer us great protection from cancer, we cannot rely on them to do the whole job. Some alterations in our diet will have to be made. What are they? An article on cancer prevention in the May 1976 issue of *Family Health* succinctly sums them up: "First of all, eat less fat, particularly beef fat: substitute chicken and fish for those endless hamburgers, a small steak for a large one. Eat more fresh fruits and vegetables. . . . Most importantly, avoid highly refined grains and cereals. . . . Learn to eat whole wheat bread and other unrefined cereal products."

Fish makes an excellent substitute for meat. It is not only generally lower in fat, but it is often a storehouse for selenium, nucleic acid, and other valuable ingredients. Three inexpensive and easily available types of fish are especially recommended. They are sardines, which are high in nucleic acid; herring, which is high in zinc; and tuna, which is a fairly good provider of selenium. Tuna fish is a favorite food of nutritionist Jean Mayer, who chaired a presidential commission on nutrition. However, when using sardines and tuna fish, you would do well to wash them in water first to get rid of the oil and some of the salt that have been added to them.

White flour is undoubtedly another cancer catalyst. It is flour that has been stripped of most of its fiber, most of its magnesium, most of its vitamin E, and much of its zinc and selenium. Other valuable nutrients have also been lost in processing. When it has been bleached with chlorine dioxide it becomes doubly damaging, for not only has it lost most of its antioxidant vitamin E, but it has now been dosed with an oxidant as well. Oxidants, don't forget, are believed to make us age faster than we should and to foster, or at least facilitate, the development of cancer.

Commercial whole wheat bread is not the best substitute for white bread, since commercial whole wheat, as a glance at the list of contents on the label will show, still contains much white flour as well. (You will note, when reading the contents, that they often include caramel coloring designed to make the bread look darker than it ordinarily would be.) However, if bread made completely from whole wheat is not available to you or is too expensive, then use the commercial whole wheat. It is far better than white bread. Rye bread is also to be preferred to white bread, though rye flour contains less of the valuable nutrients found in whole wheat.

Brown rice and potatoes constitute other valuable components of the anticancer diet. Brown rice is rich in B vitamins and fiber. Potatoes contain some vitamins and some minerals as well. Both are very low in sodium, while the peel of potatoes is very rich in potassium.

You may be wondering if consuming all these carbohydrates won't create weight problems? The answer is no. As a matter of fact, you will tend to lose weight. Several studies have shown that most people actually shed excess pounds on high-bread diets, at least when the bread comes from whole grain flour. In one experiment, six people who were given a diet high in whole grain bread but allowed to eat all they wanted of anything else automatically ended up consuming 100 calories less per day. At Michigan State University, Dr. Olaf Mickelson placed students on a similar diet: plenty of whole grain bread plus as much as they wanted of other foods. Those who ate more than seven slices a day lost nearly six pounds in seven weeks.

Potatoes are widely believed to be fattening, but the figures indicate otherwise. A baked potato contains 93 calories, while a mashed potato, even with milk added, provides only 65. A 3½-ounce steak, even if it is cut fairly lean, can pump over 400 calories into your system. As for brown rice, well, just look at the Chinese or Japanese who customarily remain quite slender on diets consisting largely of rice.

The fact is that whole grains, rice, especially brown rice, and potatoes are what are sometimes called complex carbohydrates. As opposed to the simple carbohydrates, such as white flour, they tend, besides providing us with much more nourishment, to give us a filled-up feeling.

The writer of the article in Family Health says elsewhere in his article, "Fat helps promote the action of carcinogenic chemicals." We saw in our discussion that a research physician working for the National Cancer Institute told that fat tends to upset the hormonal balance. Further confirmation of this point is provided by Dr. Ernst Wynder, president of the American Health Federation and by Dr. Michael J. Hill of the Central Public Laboratory in London. Dr. Hill believes that certain bacteria in the colon change cholesterol and bile acids into estrogenlike carcinogens, and these carcinogens make their way to estrogen-receptive organs such as the breast or ovary.

The average American now consumes 157 grams or nearly six ounces of fat a day. The people in the three long-life and nearly cancer-free regions that we have frequently used for comparison consume much less. The south Russian group eat only 40 to 60 grams a day, the Pakistani group ingest a mere 36 grams a day, while the Ecuadorian group get by on a measly 12 to 19 grams of fat a day. Thus, the average inhabitant of even the region where the most fat is consumed eats, on the average, only about one-quarter as much fat as the average American.

Beef is easily the most dangerous of meats as the *Family Health* writer seems to indicate. Except for liver and possibly other beef organs, such as kidneys, it should be eaten sparingly. Chicken is probably the safest and most wholesome meat since it is low in fat and since the darker meat of the chicken contains a good deal of nucleic acid.

Legumes, such as beans and peas, are another type of food that belong high on the anticancer menu. In general, they are high-potassium, low-sodium, and fibrous foods. Lentil, pinto, and gazebo beans are especially recommended for they not only contain many minerals and some vitamins, but also furnish goodly amounts of nucleic acid. Legumes also yield protein, and while we should not consume too much protein, we should, of course, make sure that we do not become protein-deficient. Too little protein, while it may spare us from cancer, can give us other problems.

It goes without saying that we should restrict our intake of salt and sugar. Put some healthful herbs, such as sage, thyme, tarragon, and basil, on your table and use them instead of salt. After you get used to them, you will find that substituting them for salt actually increases the flavor of most foods. Don't forget that the French use very little salt in their cooking, yet many gourmets consider French cuisine to be the most flavorsome in the world.

Sugar often presents an even greater problem, since the

average American currently derives about 20 percent of his calories from this source. Honey often makes an excellent substitute. It not only contains many healthful and apparently cancer-protecting nutrients, but it also, per calorie consumed, provides more sweetness. Thus, you can obtain the same degree of sweetness from a lesser amount of honey. Furthermore, while many of us can consume sugar-based products almost indefinitely, we find that those made of honey satiate our sweetness demands much more rapidly.

Molasses can also take the place of sugar. It contains calcium, iron, and most of the B vitamins, and like honey it tends to slake our desire for something sweet much more effectively than refined sugar. Grapes, dates, and figs also supply sweetness in a better form than refined sugar. Finally, if you must use sugar, then try to use dark brown or raw sugar. These at least contain some mineral salts and do less damage to the system. As noted earlier, tests at the Dartmouth Medical School's trace mineral laboratory have shown that while refined white sugar tends to deplete the body's supply of chromium, dark brown sugar, along with honey and molasses, tends to increase chromium in the body.

Because canned goods nearly always contain sugar and salt, and because canned food often loses some of its healthful properties, we should prefer fresh foods instead. However, not all of us can or would want to give up canned foods completely. There are ways of transforming many canned foods into much more nutritious, as well as much more appetizing, table fare.

For example, chili con carne can be purchased in a can, and while it will have some sugar, some salt, and possibly some other undesirable substances added to it, nevertheless the chili and the beans themselves are nourishing foods. My wife and I add chopped onions, garlic, and brewer's yeast to the chile, putting in the yeast just before we take it off the stove so as to protect the yeast from too much exposure to heat. Then we sprinkle dill over it and put it on some whole grain bread or brown rice or some extra lean hamburger. The result is an inexpensive, easy-to-prepare, generally nutritious, and most appetizing meal.

Italian canned soups also lend themselves to such embellishment, for they generally contain, in contrast to American-style canned soups, little or no added salt or sugar. We take lentil soups, for example, and add to it the tops of any vegetables we have in the refrigerator, plus yeast, garlic, and other healthful ingredients. The soup, which is quite thick to begin with, can be poured over brown rice or eaten by itself. In either case, the result is a nutritious, appetizing, and inexpensive meal.

Spaghetti can also be transformed into a most nutritious meal, especially if whole wheat spaghetti is used. Brewer's yeast, as well as lots of onions and garlic can be used in the sauce to make the resulting dish as beneficial for our bodies as it is pleasing to our palates.

Many casserole dishes, especially if they are made from healthful things, such as tuna fish or lentils, can be made more tasty and more cancer-preventive through nutritional supplementation. Milk shakes can be made with carob powder in place of chocolate plus a spoonful of yeast, the yolk of an egg, honey, and even a banana. Cereals, perhaps more than anything else can be turned into treasure houses of nourishment with the addition of such foods as brewer's yeast, wheat germ, sesame seeds, bananas, and raisins. Experimenting in this way can furnish a lot of fun as well as supply meals that will help protect you from cancer.

Even ordinary junk foods can be greatly improved. If you order a sub, make it a tuna fish sub with hot peppers and onions as well as lettuce and tomato. If a pizza, then order it with onions or mushrooms or, preferably, both. And if you must eat a chocolate bar, then make sure it is the kind with almonds. There are always ways of minimizing the damage, even when you can't contribute to health.

Hamburgers, that mainstay of the American diet, are best eaten rarely. Charcoal-broiled hamburgers are likely to contain less fat. Hot dogs are best avoided altogether. They are filled with fat and all kinds of obnoxious flavoring and coloring agents. A hot dog, by the way, contains two-and-a-half times the calories of a slice of bread. Take a meal of hot dogs, white rolls, and Cokes, and you've got a meal fit for facilitating the development of cancer.

Try to eat more fresh vegetables and fruit, urges *Family Health*, and this too is good advice. The best vegetables are undoubtedly garlic, onions, mushrooms, hot red peppers, and asparagus, but most all vegetables are beneficial. If you are worried that garlic will give you bad breath, then chew a piece of parsley afterward. As an alternative, take garlic oil tablets or garlic and parsley tablets, both of which are sold in health food stores. Also, learn to use horseradish. It can be mixed in with tuna fish, applied directly to fish or meat, or simply spread on a piece of bread.

By all means eat eggs, unless you are one of the rare individuals who cannot metabolize them. Eggs are complete organisms containing everything necessary for the formation of a baby chick. They are thus one of the most healthful foods available at your supermarket. Oysters, clams, yeast, and mushrooms fall somewhat in the same category. They, too, may be generously consumed.

What about organic food, that is, food grown without the use of chemical fertilizers and pesticides? It is obviously to be preferred. However, it tends to be somewhat expensive and often unavailable. Many times it has been transported long distances, and sometimes it does not appear too appetizing when it shows up on the stands. But, some organic food can and should be consumed, at least now and then, to remove or dilute whatever effects the chemicals from regular food may have produced on our systems.

Raw food is another important feature of the anticancer diet. We know that cooking tends to destroy or diminish many of the vitamins and at least one important mineral, magnesium, in food. It also does away with various enzymes and possibly other important ingredients. Finally, cooked food evokes a reaction in our bodies that indicates that the human system finds it harmful. Cooked food, so research has revealed, causes our white cell count to go up. In other words, the human body responds to such food in the same manner as it responds to an infection!

This strange and suspicious response can be overcome if one eats raw food prior to a meal. The cooked food, so tests have shown, then does not trigger such a response from our immunization system. Another benefit from beginning the meal with raw food, such as a salad, is that it usually consists of more roughage than the cooked portion of the meal and will, therefore, help us achieve a filled-up feeling sooner. As a result, we may find it easier not to eat so much.

In thinking about raw food, do not forget nuts and seeds. They usually provide lots of fiber, many minerals and vitamins, and some protein and unsaturated fat as well. Pumpkin seeds, sunflower seeds, and sesame seeds are especially nutritious, but even more common kinds, such as peanuts, have much to offer. Such fruits as dried apricots, dried prunes, and raisins, are also valuable. My wife frequently puts on the table a dish containing a mixture of pumpkin seeds, sunflower seeds, roasted soybeans, and raisins, and our family dips into it quite freely for snacks.

For beverages, try substituting fruit juices, including apple juice, for soft drinks and try substituting herbal teas, especially ginseng, for at least some of the regular tea and coffee in your diet. Buttermilk, is also helpful, as, of course, is yogurt.

Do not forget to extend the benefits of the anticancer diet to the children in your life as well. Although cancer strikes most frequently at older people, it attacks youngsters as well. It is, as a matter of fact, after accidents, the second greatest killer of children. More importantly, childhood is the time when eating habits are first formed and when the cornerstones of health are put in place. Try to make sure the proper cornerstones of health are laid in the children you have contact with. Substitute nuts and seeds, peanuts and popcorn, raisins and other dried fruits for the sugar so many adults willingly allow their youngsters to consume.

Don't forget that the benefits of the anticancer diet and life-style extend far beyond the area of cancer protection itself. In adopting an anticancer regimen you will, in all likelihood, experience fewer colds, suffer less trouble from constipation and related problems (such as hemorrhoids), find it easier to control your weight, and lead a longer and more vigorous life.

The anticancer diet, as you may have already noted, will also tend to protect you from heart disease. Its low-sodium, high-potassium base, its restrictions on meat and fat, and its encouragement to eat such foods as fish, especially sardines, garlic, onions, apples, mushrooms, and yogurt should all help your heart to stay healthy.

If Cancer Strikes

The anticancer program outlined in the pages of this book will most probably keep you cancer-free. Certainly evidence strongly suggests that it will. But 100 percent protection cannot be guaranteed. If you have been unable to follow all of its admonitions, or if you have already lived a lifetime on a substantially different regimen, or if you have become overly exposed to cancer-causing substances, or even if you have a greatly weakened immunization system, it may still be possible for you to contract cancer.

What should you do if this occurs? Obviously, you must seek treatment and follow your doctor's orders. But with his or her permission, you should greatly step up your adherence to the anticancer regimen. Cut out all salt and all meat and greatly increase your consumption of raw fruits, vegetables, and whole grains. Garlic, onions, mushrooms, and especially asparagus should be eaten daily. Honey, pollen, yogurt, brewer's yeast, and desiccated liver should also be on your daily menu. Make sure the honey is raw and has not been heated. (Some brands of honey list themselves as "uncooked," but uncooked is not the same as unheated.) Try to eat organic food. Drink ginseng tea or take it in tablet form every day (the Siberian variety seems most effective). Increase your consumption of vitamins, kelp, magnesium, and other supplements.

Many cancer patients lose their appetite for food. If this happens to you, then force yourself to overcome it. Your immunization system still exists, but it needs proper nourishment to do its job.

If you smoke, and if your doctor has *not* told you to give it up, then continue smoking. Giving up smoking can place a person under substantial stress before the habit is completely broken. You certainly do not need any further stress if you have cancer. Indeed, a relaxed and confident attitude can help your immunization system greatly, as Dr. Simonton has shown.

Remaining confident and calm in the face of a serious and growing cancer seems impossible and even idiotic. But almost any seasoned cancer specialist can tell of cases where an ordinarily fatal case of cancer failed to fulfill its gloomy prognosis and the patient lived. Medical miracles do occur, and by pursuing the proper anticancer program you can, at least somewhat, increase the possibility that one will occur in your case.

How to Treat Your Doctor

A study at the Harvard Medical School once showed that the average doctor at the school knew just a little more nutrition than the average secretary at the school. That is, unless the secretary was overweight. If she was, then she was likely to know just a bit more about nutrition than the average doctor. If this reflects the extent of nutritional knowledge among doctors at the nation's most prestigious medical school, one can imagine how much the typical practicing physician knows about the subject.

For this reason and for some others that we will examine shortly, your doctor will probably give the nutritional approach little credence. Obviously, if he does feel it to be of some value, he will mention it himself. If you were to raise the subject and he were to admit its validity, then he would be admitting that he had not told you something that you ought to know. It goes without saying that few doctors will wish to make such an admission. Their professional esteem and ego are at stake.

All of this means that you must broach the question of nutritional therapy with your doctor cautiously. You know that your doctor is a highly trained person who knows more about your system than anyone else. You certainly do not want to do anything that he has sound reasons for disapproving. Yet, you do wish to avail yourself of the help that nutrition can provide. What do you do?

The answer, in a nutshell, is to *seek your doctor's permission but not necessarily his approval.* In other words, don't ask him if the anticancer regimen is going to do you any good; ask him, rather, whether it is going to do you any harm. If he cannot offer you any medical reason why it should do you any harm, then adopt it.

Sometimes, you may find it necessary to soothe his ego first or to make sure that he holds no grudges against you for pursuing an approach that he has not recommended. You can do this in a number of ways. For example, you might tell him that you have heard about the anticancer diet, that you realize it probably will do you no particular good (otherwise he would have recommended it himself), but that you promised a friend or a loved one that you would try it. Does he have any objection?

If your doctor does have a valid objection—and I mean an objection based upon one or more specific and stated reasons, not just some general antipathy to "nutrition nuts"—then by all means do what he says. If you have some doubt about the validity of his objections, then get another doctor. In no case should you ever disobey a doctor's advice as long as he can give distinctly medical reasons for it.

The real tragedy, however, is that one sometimes has to fall back upon such stratagems in dealing with one's doctor. Why should this ever be necessary? Why are doctors so ignorant of, and so hostile or at least antipathetic to, nutritional approaches?

The problem begins in medical school. Most of these schools omit nutrition from their curriculum. What is still worse, they provide a type of training that focuses on the use of drugs and surgery to cure ailments, not on the use of proper health habits to prevent them. "Medical education," writes Dr. Roger Williams, "has neglected to perform a refined study of nutrition in all its aspects and has diverted attention away from the most promising means of controlling cancer. That avenue is the nutritional approach. . . ."

The physician takes the education and habits that he learned in medical school into his daily practice. As time goes by, they become more deeply ingrained. What's more, he often becomes too busy to read such nutritional information as may come his way in medical journals. Instead, he relies too heavily on the brochures from the drug companies and on spiels from their salesmen to keep them up to date on recent developments.

To adopt a nutritional approach to the problems of disease would consequently require that most physicians make a complete change in their orientation to medicine. And change has never come easily to the medical profession. Fifty years after William Harvey conclusively demonstrated that the blood circulates through the body, many of his medical colleagues still refused to believe it. The great Austrian physician Semmelweis literally went insane in his feverish, but largely futile, efforts to get his fellow doctors to wash their hands before delivering children. Pasteur could elicit almost no medical support for his microbe theories. He had to wait for another generation of doctors to appear on the scene before he was able to persuade the profession to accept his findings. A mere generation ago, Louis Pillemer, a young professor at Yale, made one of the important discoveries regarding the immunization theory—he spotted a new substance in the blood that was not an antibody but could nevertheless act as one—only to find his discovery greeted by derision. He ended up killing himself.

Yes, he who would persuade the medical profession to change its mind has his work cut out for him. Of course, reluctance and resistance toward change is not limited to doctors. Most of us balk at new ideas that seem to contradict our learning and experience. Adelle Davis, for example, refused to reexamine any of her nutritional policies when she was dying of cancer. On the contrary, she felt that she had become susceptible to malignancy because she had not practiced her ideas faithfully enough.

A doctor, however, has an additional reason for resisting the new nutritional approach to medicine and health. This approach not only challenges his education and training, but also challenges his professional status and his pocketbook.

The American physician is probably the most highly trained professional man in the world. Medical school is probably the most demanding of all graduate schools, and American medical schools, so it seems, are the most demanding of all. Thus a medical doctor in this country enjoys great prestige and the perquisites that go with it.

Nutritional medicine does not make use of all this hard-earned education. Nutritional approaches are essentially simple ones. In most cases they do not even require the right to write a prescription. They thus threaten the physician's professional prestige and esteem. You may remember the disgusted and dismayed reaction of one of the cancer specialists who were treating young Johnny Gunther when Dr. Gerson came on the scene: "If this thing works, we can chuck millions of dollars worth of expensive equipment and start cooking carrots in a pot."

Look at it another way. Doctors Jonas Salk and Albert Sabin received praise and renown for discovering the respective vaccines that bear their names. But Dr. Klenner, who has found that vitamin C can also stave off, and in some cases at least, cure infantile paralysis, remains largely unknown to the general public. If a doctor, aware not only of Klenner's work, but also of Jungeblut's experiment in preventing polio in monkeys through vitamin C, had successfully used the vitamin as a preventive during the New England polio epidemic of the mid-1950s, where would this have gotten him? Not very far. No vaccine would bear his name and no patent would be earning royalties.

The subject of royalties brings us to another and possibly greater reason for modern medicine's antipathy to, and avoidance of, nutritional measures. American medicine is largely curative, not preventive, and American doctors are largely concerned with curing illness, not maintaining health; the entire reward system is based upon this approach. As Dr. Gio Gori of the National Cancer Institute has pointed out, "The problem with 'prevention' is that it does not produce revenues. No health plan reimburses a physician or a hospital for preventing a disease." The fact is that if we kept ourselves in top condition, most hospitals, doctors, and pharmaceutical companies would go broke. This does not mean that your doctor wants you to become ill. Of course not. But it does detract from his desire to keep you in maximum health. At best, it sets up a system that relegates health to a secondary position.

The consequences of such a system became appallingly apparent to me when I once asked a young pediatrician whether she advised mothers to breast feed their children. She was aware that such breast feeding may protect the mother from breast cancer later on and that it furnishes superior nourishment to her baby. Yet she said that neither she nor most of her fellow pediatricians pointed this out to the mothers of their young patients. When I asked why, she replied, "Well, breast feeding is harder to manage."

"What do you mean?" I asked, somewhat mystified.

"Supposing a mother calls you up in the middle of the night and complains that her breast has gone dry? These are some of the problems with managing breast feeding," she said.

"But what of the protective effect of breast feeding in terms of breast cancer? Don't you think you should at least tell the mother about this?" I continued.

"Oh, that wouldn't mean much. Most people don't worry about things that may happen to them twenty or thirty years from now."

You may think this young woman especially cold and callous, but I can assure you that she isn't. She is probably better motivated than most doctors, for she even went to

Africa for a while to provide medical care to people who enjoy little access to such service. Yet her answers vividly demonstrate how the system itself has succeeded in depriving even its more dedicated practitioners of the desire and the drive to promote, to the fullest extent possible, the health of their patients.

Toward a Healthier Future

Out of the disgruntlement and despair that our current so-called health-care system has developed, a new form of medicine is starting to emerge. It stresses prevention rather than cure, it puts nutrition before drugs, and it focuses on the patient rather than just on his illness.

This new form of health care is called *orthomolecular medicine*, an unnecessarily complicated name for what is essentially a simpler and more basic approach toward improving the nation's health. But, by whatever name it is called, it is fast gaining ground. Just a few years ago, six physicians, along with some other health professionals, formed the International Academy of Preventive Medicine. By 1976, the number of physician members had grown to around five hundred, with more of them joining all the time. In March 1976 they invited Robert Rodale, publisher of *Prevention* magazine to speak before them. Commented Rodale, "There was a time when I had trouble getting into a medical convention as a reporter." Slowly but surely, American medicine is starting to respond to the freshening currents of change.

Many of the doctors who are becoming interested in the new preventive approach are young, but some of them are not. Dr. August Daro, professor of obstetrics and gynecology at Loyola Stritch School of Medicine and the Cook County

Postgraduate School of Medicine, both in Chicago, did not start taking nutrition seriously until he was seventy. At seventy-six, he is now dispensing nutritional supplements to his patients and taking them himself. He works a very full day, starting at 5 A.M. when he takes the first of this thrice-daily batches of vitamins and minerals. (Incidentally, Dr. Daro eats two eggs every morning and sometimes two more at lunch. "I want to disprove this silly notion that you mustn't eat eggs on account of cholesterol," he told *Prevention*.)

Some of medicine's leading lights have shown up in the ranks of this new movement. For example, thirty Nobel prize winners are on the board of the Linus Pauling Institute, an institute formed to foster through research the goals of orthomolecular medicine. Meanwhile, Dr. Charles Butterworth, Jr., a prominent figure in the American Medical Association, has spoken out sharply on the woeful ignorance of most doctors and the distressing negligence of most hospitals in dealing with nutrition. In an article in the March-April 1974 issue of *Nutrition Today*, Dr. Butterworth cites cases of patients suffering debilitation, and even dying, as the result of this lack of concern. Dr. Albert Sabin has called for more research on the role that nutrition could play in the prevention of cancer. The discoverer of a famous vaccine himself, he claims that efforts to develop a similar one for cancer hold out little hope. Prevention through nutrition, says Dr. Sabin, offers the best possibility for licking this problem.

All these encouraging signs, however, have not yet sufficed to turn modern medicine around. What is needed, among other things, is a different reward system, *one that will reward health-care practitioners for promoting health rather than for treating illness.* Perhaps the best prospect for achieving this is through the increasing use of health-maintenance organizations that take care of a person's health problems on a flat fee basis. Such an organization thereby has incentive for keeping the client as healthy as possible: to hold down its own costs.

But whether it's through the use of health-maintenance organizations or through the use of other devices and approaches, the need for some change is becoming increasingly apparent. The nation is now spending nearly ten percent of its gross national product for health care, and this is affecting our entire economy. General Motors, for example, now pays out more for employee health insurance that it does for the steel to make its cars.

What makes this enormous expenditure doubly tragic is that it has not improved the nation's health all that much. A sixty-year-old man today can expect to live only about a year longer than could a sixty-year-old man in 1789. America's mortality rates for most ailments and health problems, and the country's overall longevity rate, fall below those of most Western European countries, which expend a far smaller proportion of their national income on health care.

Yes, something is clearly amiss, and this is fueling the change that is coming about in medicine. This change will eventually reduce the incidence of cancer substantially, as well as increase the nation's overall health and lengthen its average life span. But most of us cannot and should not wait. We can, and we should, start our anticancer program now.

Start yours today!

Bibliographical Notes and Comments

Chapter 1: A Peril and a Hope

Information on the development of the immunization theory comes largely from *The Body Is the Hero* by Ronald J. Glasser, M.D. (Random House, 1976). An article in the December 1976–January 1977 issue of *Modern Maturity* also contains some interesting information on how modern medicine is starting to link cancer control to the individual immunization system. Entitled "Our Bodies' Own Cancer Cures," the unsigned article discusses the work of Dr. Antonio Rottino, a cancer researcher at Saint Vincent's Hospital in New York City. Dr. Rottino has become convinced that a healthy body will overcome most cancers.

Chapter 2: The Case of Dr. Gerson

This chapter was greatly influenced by two books: *Has Dr. Max Gerson a True Cancer Cure?* by S. J. Haught (London Press, 1962) and *Death Be Not Proud* by John Gunther (Harper, 1949). The quote from Sauerbruch will be found in Haught. The famed surgeon's autobiography, *Master Surgeon*, was published in English many years ago by Thomas Y. Crowell Company but is now, regrettably, out of print.

In recent years many other cases have come to light of people curing themselves of cancer by following diets similar to those that Gerson prescribed. They include a Danish physician, the wife of a prominent American business man, and a young Malayan Chinese, all of whom have published books on their experiences. These books are *My Experiences with Living Food* by Kristine Nolfi, M.D. (Solana Health Center, n.d.), *How I Conquered Cancer Naturally* by Eydie Mae Hunsberger (Harvest House Publishers, 1976), and *How I Overcame Inoperable Cancer* by Wong Hon Sun, M.D. (Exposition Press, 1975.) Mrs. Hunsberger, the wife of the president of the U.S. Elevator Company, suffered from breast cancer as did Dr. Nolfi. Wong contracted what was diagnosed as anaplastic epidermoid carcinoma, a cancerous growth formed from the epidermal cells of a mucous membrane. The tumor was nonoperable because of its great size, and he was given no chance to survive.

In addition I have interviewed Kim Hubbard of Putney, Vermont, who also defied his doctors' prognosis by going on a Gerson-like diet and thereby conquering a severe case of bowel cancer.

Chapter 3: Toward the Glasgow Experiment

Most of the information on the general beneficial effects of vitamin C can be found in articles on this subject in *Prevention*, June 1973; November 1974; January 1975; and September 1976; and in *Nature's Way*, July 1974. More professional readers may wish to consult Dr. Frederick Klenner's own publications. They include "The Use of Vitamin C as an Antibiotic," *Journal of Applied Nutrition* 6 (1953): 247; "Massive Doses of Vitamin C and Virus Diseases," *Southern Medicine and Surgery* 110 (1951): 101; "The Vitamin Treatment for Acute Poliomyelitis," *Southern Medicine* 114 (1952): 194; "Virus Pneumonia and Its Treatment With Vitamin C," *Southern Medicine* 110 (1948): 36. Dr. Williamson recounts her experience in administering vitamin C to ther snake-bitten dog in a letter to *Prevention*, January 1975.

Linus Pauling's 1970 book, *Vitamin C and the Common Cold*, was first published by W. H. Freeman and Company and reprinted the following year in paperback by Bantam. However, in 1976 Dr. Pauling published a new book entitled *Vitamin C, the Common Cold and the Flu*. In this work, he presented still more evidence of the effectiveness of vitamin C in combating viral infections while answering critics of his earlier work (this new book was also published by W. H. Freeman).

The famed Toronto study on this subject was first published in the *Canadian Medical Association Journal* of April 5, 1975, but has been summarized extensively elsewhere. The *New York Times* of October 13, 1974, carries a news item reporting it, along with some of the other studies cited in this book.

The study in Scotland by Doctors Charleston and Clegg was reported in the June 24, 1976, *Lancet*; Dr. Coulehan's study was reported by him at a symposium in Stanford, California, on August 7, 1973. An Associated Press dispatch of that date summing up his results appeared in newspapers throughout the country.

Dr. Michael Halberstam's article appeared in The *New York Times Magazine*, March 17, 1974. The NIH study seeking to refute claims of vitamin C's effectiveness in cold prevention was reported in the *Journal of the American Medical Association* of March 10, 1975.

One further note regarding antisupernutritionist Dr. Frederick Stare may be of interest. In 1976 he was given an award by the National Confectionery Makers Association. This is the national organization of candy makers.

For data on the two British studies concerning vitamin C and the elderly see the *British Medical Journal,* May 17, 1969; the *American Journal of Clinical Nutrition,* February 27, 1974; and *Prevention*, July 1974. For data on the danger of scurvy to cancer patients, see *Prevention*, June 1975.

The work of the University of Nebraska Medical Center on nitrites, cancer, and vitamin C was reported in the June 7, 1972, *Science*. The findings of the Chinese in this field were covered in the *Chinese Medical Journal*, May 1975. Dr. Schlegal's discoveries regarding vitamin C and bladder cancer can be found in the *Medical World News*, June 21, 1968. For a more comprehensive account see the article by him and his associates in the *Journal of Urology*, February 1970. Dr. Cheraskin's remarks are reported by Dr. Carlton Fredericks in his column in *Prevention*, June 1976.

As noted in the text, the results of the Scottish experiment in using vitamin C against cancer can be found in the October 1976 *Proceedings of the National Academy of Sciences*. However, Pauling briefly reviews much of this material in his 1976 book cited earlier. Articles on this important experiment also appeared in July 1975, November 1975, and

January 1977 issues of *Prevention*. Also see an interview with Linus Pauling in the January 1977 *Let's Live*.

Dr. Irwin Stone's scrupulously documented book *The Healing Factor: Vitamin C Against Disease* (Grosset & Dunlap, 1971) is probably the most complete work published up to that time on the role of this vitamin in human health. Chapter 15 deals with cancer and deserves the close attention of all those seriously concerned with dealing with this disease. The source for the case of the elderly leukemiac cited by Stone is given as *Medical Times* (Manhasset) 82 (1954).

The article cited by Dr. Charles E. Butterworth, Jr., appeared in the *American Journal of Clinical Nutrition*, August 1974. In this article, Dr. Butterworth discusses not only the role of vitamin C in preventing heart disease but the role of another controversial compound as well. This second heart-protecting nutriment is a compound called lecithin. We examine it briefly in the discussion of eggs in the diet in Chapter 9.

Two other items are also worthy of note. One is an article entitled "Boost Your Immunity with Vitamin C," which appeared in *Prevention* of May 1977. In this article, Benjamin Siegel, Ph.D., of the University of Oregon Health Sciences Center outlined, in an interview, his research showing how vitamin C actually managed to bolster the body's immunization system. The second article, "Vitamin C as a Cold Pill," appeared in the January 1977 issue of *Let's Live*. It was authored by B. F. Hart, M.D., and Anne L. Hendricks, M.D., two practicing physicians from Fort Lauderdale, Florida. Doctors Hart and Hendricks claim that "Vitamin C, *when given in adequate doses*, enables the body defenses to destroy viruses of all classes impartially." And, although a few people cannot tolerate it, "we know of no instance where Vitamin C has caused a serious side effect or undesired sequel."

Chapter 4: The A B E's of Cancer Prevention

The research done by Kagan and Kaiser on vitamin A was reported in the *Journal of Nutrition* 57, number 2 (1955). Dr. Odens's work with the vitamin first came to light in an article he wrote for the December 1967 issue of the German medical publication *Vitalstoffe*. For Dr. Chernov's article see *The American Journal of Surgery* 122 (1972), and for a write-up on Dr. Cohen's finding see *Medical World News,* December 14, 1973. *Prevention,* May 1976, carried a summary of Dr. Seifter's findings.

Tannock's early work was published in the *Journal of the National Cancer Institute* 48 (1942). A good account of Dr. Saffiotti's 1968 paper can be found in *Prevention* of April 1972. Dr. Shamberger published his findings in the September 1971 *Journal of the National Cancer Institute.* The Norwegian study appeared in the *International Journal of Cancer* 15 (1975).

There have been reports of numerous other studies linking vitamin A with cancer. The February 1974 *Let's Live* said that the *National Institute of Allergy and Infectious Disease* had found vitamin A to increase measurably the resistance of mice to cancer cells. On November 2, 1975, the *Boston Globe* carried a story saying that experimenters at MIT had found that many rats developed colon cancer once deprived of the vitamin. In 1977 the National Cancer Institute, enheartened by its own tests, asked the Food and Drug Administration for permission to test the vitamin as a preventive measure on humans with high risk of contracting cancer of the bladder, breast, and uterus.

The report on autopsies showing that up to 37 percent of Americans may be vitamin A–deficient was published in the March 1972 issue of the *American Journal of Clinical Nutrition*. For further information on HEW's ten-state survey, see *Prevention*, of February 1973. Judging from a report in the *Journal of the Canadian Medical Association* of December 13, 1969, Canada appears to be suffering from the same problem.

One final item regarding vitamin A may be of interest. Some years ago, Dr. Henry C. Sherman of Columbia University found that boosting substantially the amounts of vitamin A in diets of laboratory animals increased average longevity 10 percent in the males and 12 percent in the females.

The early suggestive work on B vitamins and cancer control done by the New York Skin and Cancer Hospital and at a Canadian medical school are cited by Carlton Fredericks and Herbert Bailey in their book *Food Facts and Fallacies* (Arco, 1965). The article in the *American Journal of Surgery* on brewer's yeast and mouth cancer was authored by Hayes Martin, M.D., and Everett Koop, M.D. For the effects of inositol, see *Proceedings of the Society for Experimental Biological Medicine* 54 (1943) and *Journal of Urology* 59 (1948).

Dr. Williams's book, *Nutrition Against Disease*, is available in paperback (Bantam, 1971). Dr. Mount's work is reported in *Body, Mind and the B Vitamins* by Ruth Adams and Frank Murray, with a foreword by Abram Hoffer, M.D. (Larchmont, 1974). The report on niacinamide can be found in the February 1, 1972, issue of *Biochemistry*, which is published by the American Chemical Society.

The research on PABA and skin cancer was reported in the *New England Journal of Medicine*, June 26, 1969. Dr. Axlerod's quote comes from *Prevention*, April, 1972: Dr. Newberne's conclusions were cited in *Science News*, August 17, 1974; and Dr. Warburg's list of anticancer B vitamins was mentioned in the March, 1973, *Prevention*.

The quote from *Medical Letter* regarding vitamin E and the discovery by the National Research Council are from Richard A. Passwater's "The Great Vitamin E Controversy" in the May 1974 issue of *Prevention*. Passwater is a biochemist who has intensively studied vitamin E. His article contains much other recent research on this still not very well known vitamin.

Doctors Ayres and Mihan first reported their work in the *Journal of the American Medical Association*, January 10, 1972, and later in the *Southern Medical Journal*, November, 1974. Bailey's book, *Your Key to a Healthy Heart,* was published by Chilton Books in 1965. Much has been written about, and by, the Shute brothers. One short book that deals with their work and the work of others in this field is *Vitamin E, Wonder Worker of the 70's?* by Ruth Adams and Frank Murray (1971). It is available in paperback from Larchmont Books and carries a foreword by Dr. Evan Shute.

Dr. Ochsner's letter was published in the *New England Journal of Medicine* of July 23, 1964. Also see his "Preventing and Treating Venous Thrombosis" in *Postgraduate Medicine*, July 1968. He is the founder of an internationally renown clinic that bears his name.

Another report on vitamin E and air pollution, besides the one cited in the text, was published in *Nutrition Reports International*, June 1975. The research conducted by Doctors Black and Lo at Baylor was published in *Nature*, December 21–28, 1973. And the experiments carried out at the Cleveland Clinic Foundation on anti-oxidants and cell damage were published in the May 1973 *Proceedings of the National Academy of Sciences.*

Dr. Ayres's observation about vitamin E and progeria appeared in a communication to the *Journal of the American Medical Association* of March 25, 1974. For reports on Dr.

Harmon's work on vitamin E and longevity and on the California experiment regarding human lung tissue, see Taub's article in *Prevention*, February 1975.

Other studies using laboratory animals indicate that vitamin E helps ulcers to heal (see *American Journal of Clinical Nutrition*, September 1972) and strengthens the immunization system. Finally, a personal experience may be of some relevance. Prior to taking vitamin E, I had been increasingly feeling the need to elevate my feet and legs while sitting down. It had reached the point where I could not sit at a desk for more than fifteen minutes without wanting desperately to put my feet up. However, shortly after I started to take vitamin E, this need began to quickly diminish.

Chapter 5: Minerals That Help You Resist Cancer

Information on Dr. Delbert and magnesium comes from chapter 13 of *Gesund Sein!* by Jean Palaiseul (Zurich: Albert Muller Verlag, 1973). This is a most interesting book, which covers several unconventional methods of maintaining health and longevity. It is available in French, under the title *Tous les espoirs de guerir* (Paris: Robert Laffont S.A.), but not, unfortunately, in English. The data concerning French studies of magnesium in the soil and cancer is taken largely from *Magnesium, the Nutrient that Could Change Your Life* by J. I. Rodale (Pyramid, 1968).

Dr. Selye's work with magnesium and stress was written up in an article on this mighty mineral in the April 1973 *Prevention*. For deficiency of magnesium and heart attack victims, see *Medical Tribune*, September 21, 1970. *Lancet* of August 1973 reports a similar finding. The January 20, 1973, issue of *Lancet* presents material concerning hard water versus soft water in relation to heart attacks, and the April 1973 issue of *Engineering Digest* also reports research on this point. Those who wish more information regarding the relationship between magnesium and the heart should consult the February 22, 1965, *Journal of the American Medical Association* and the June 1964 *American Journal of Clinical Nutrition* for data concerning magnesium's ability to act against high blood pressure.

The Chicago experiment exploring magnesium and leukemia was reported in the March 27, 1967, *Journal of the American Medical Association*. Dr. Hass's subsequent interview with *Prevention* took place in that magazine's July 1975 issue. I have also heard of an interesting discovery made in Poland regarding this relationship. It seems that cattle in one section of the country occasionally come down with leukemia but cattle in the rest of the country almost never do. The former section, so it seems, lies in the part of Poland that once belonged to Germany. Scientists have opined that because its soil was once subject to the more intensive cultivation of the German farmers, it is now somewhat depleted of magnesium. Hence, cattle who graze it become more subject to leukemia.

The *Journal of Nutrition* reported in June 1975 on the Iowa State University study. Dr. Mease's findings are described in a letter he published in *Lancet*, September 7, 1974. *Prevention's* interview with Dr. Rubin was published in July 1976. Dr. Seelig's comments can be found in the June 1964 *American Journal of Clinical Nutrition;* Dr. Williams's comments are from *Nutrition Against Disease.*

A good article summarizing Dr. Schwarz's work with selenium appeared in *Prevention* of August 1976. The study by the Cleveland Clinic Foundation was written up in the June 27, 1973, *Medical Tribune.* Also see *Clinical Laboratory Science* 2 (1971) and *Nutrition Reviews*, March 1970. Dr. Martin's comments in *Prevention* were published in July 1975.

Selenium, it should be noted, has also been found helpful to the heart. In his book *Supernutrition* (Dial Press, 1975) Richard A. Passwater cites various studies showing how selenium and vitamin E can work together to alleviate angina and related problems.

A comprehensive summary of Dr. Eskin's work on iodine and breast cancer can be found in *Transactions of the New York Academy of Sciences*, December 1970.

Dr. Pfeiffer discusses zinc and other minerals in his book *Mental and Elemental Nutrients, a Physician's Guide to Nutrition and Health Care* (Keats Publishing Co., 1976). Dr. Shroeder's landmark work covering zinc and other trace minerals is *The Trace Elements and Man* (Devin-Adair, 1973). Dr. Oberlas was interviewed by *Prevention* editor Robert Rodale in the magazine's September 1973 issue. This was part of an interesting and informative series on the trace mineral that the health magazine ran that year. Another and more indirect relationship between zinc and cancer can be found in a study conducted by researchers from the Washington, D.C., Veterans Administration Hospital and the National Institutes of Health. They found that a zinc deficiency makes any existing deficiency of vitamin A worse.

Here are some other items of interest about zinc. An experiment at the University of Colorado Medical Center showed that infants given zinc supplementation over a six-month period were roughly 10 percent taller and heavier than another group fed the same diet without the extra zinc. Doctors at the Uppsala University Medical School in Sweden have found that teenagers suffering from acne can reduce it by up to 85 percent through taking zinc supplements. And the February 7, 1977, *Medical World News* carried the story of a Saint Louis study showing that a group of men suffering from chronic prostatitis had only one-ninth as much zinc in their prostatic fluid as did another group of men who were free of the ailment. (Giving the prostatitis sufferers oral zinc supplements increased the amount of the mineral in their blood but not, unfortunately, in their prostatic fluid.)

The material on chromium comes mostly from Dr. Schroeder's previously cited book. The June 1977 issue of *Prevention* contains an informative article on the role chromium can play in the management of diabetes.

Dr. John Berg's remarks on molybdenum are reported in Adams and Murray's *Minerals*. Doctor DiCyan's book was published by Simon and Shuster in 1972. The Glasgow survey on potassium was published in the March 1, 1969, *Geriatric Focus*.

Chapter 6: Foods for the Fight

For a write-up of Dr. Szent-Gyorgyi's work on liver and cancer control, which includes an interview with the esteemed physician-scientist, see *Prevention*, November 1972.

Dr. Burkitt's findings regarding fiber were presented at a cancer conference in San Diego in January 1971. *Medical World News* carried a report on his remarks in its January 29, 1971, edition. On June 29, 1971, the *British Medical Journal* carried an article by Dr. Burkitt and another British physician on the same subject. The report from the National Cancer Institute can be found in the July 1975 edition of its journal. Dr. Reuben's book, *The Save-Your-Life Diet* (1976), is available in paperback from Ballantine Books.

For reports on garlic's abilities to protect the heart and promote vascular health see *Lancet* of December 29, 1973, and May 31, 1975. For other reports on garlic's far-ranging medicinal powers see *Medical Record*, June 4, 1971; *The German Medical Monthly,* March 1950; *Science Digest*, August 1971; *Today's Health*, November 1971. Actually scientific studies on garlic's medical might go back to the early 1920s.

Jane Kinderlehrer summarizes some of the research done on mushrooms in the March 1973 *Prevention*. For a documented summary of the healthful effects of yogurt see *Health Foods* by Ruth Adams and Frank Murray, with a foreword by S. Marshall Fram, M.D. (Larchmont, 1975). Also see "Of Course, There Are Helpful Germs" in *Nature's Way*, May 1975. Dr. Mann's discoveries concerning yogurt and cholesterol control were published in the May 1974 *American Journal of Clinical Nutrition*.

It should be pointed out that yogurt is by no means the only source of *Lactobacillus* culture. Buttermilk also contains it. And in 1977 several dairies began marketing a new type of milk containing *Lactobacillus* culture but tasting like ordinary nonfat milk. This new and welcome dairy product is the result of a new process by which *Lactobacillus* can be added to milk without affecting its taste.

Lactobacillus is also available in other forms. Naturally fermented sauerkraut provides it as do some fermented grains and juices. Apple cider vinegar, used in rural Vermont as a general folk remedy, also contains it. It is interesting to note in this connection that the long-living people in south Russia eat a lot of pickled food. Presumably, the type of vinegar they use for pickling provides additional *Lactobacillus* beyond what they obtain in their buttermilk.

A. J. P. Taylor's biography of Bismarck was first published by Alfred A. Knopf in 1955. It was reissued in paperback by Random House in 1967. Other Bismarck biographies make similar observations regarding the effects of the Schweringen diet. Dr. Frank's book was issued by Dial Press in 1976. Dr. Kugler's laudatory comments on Frank's work are contained in Kugler's interesting book *Slowing Down the Aging Process* (Pyramid, 1973). I have also seen an advertisement for a nucleic acid supplement called Ribomins that quotes a Clark, New Jersey, physician, Dr. V. H. Raimo, as saying that such supplements have given him much more energy.

Lutz's claims regarding asparagus were made in a lengthy letter published in the February 1974 issue of *Prevention*. Caillas's study on beekeepers and cancer was reported in his book *Gagnez 20 ans de vie grace aux abeilles* (Paris: Editions de la Penesée Moderne, 1971). Dr. Jarvis's study is covered in his book *Arthritis and Folk Medicine* (Holt, Rhinehart and Winston, 1960). Dr. Sackett's experiments are reported in *Honey and Your Health* by Bodog F. Beck, M.D., and Dorée Smedley (Dodd, Mead and Co., 1944). Dr. Blomfield's letter appeared in the *Journal of American Medical Association* on May 7, 1973. Professor Tsitsin's study of beekeeper longevity in the Soviet Union was reported in *The Bee Journal* of April 1946.

The pollen tablets taken by the nutritionally oriented American physician to cure his prostatitis came from Sweden. American pollen tablets do not work as well. (It's not that the pollen itself is so different but that the process of making it into tablets is.) Nevertheless, American pollen tablets, if consumed in sufficient quantities (at least four a day), often afford some relief. Vitamin C, wheat germ oil, along with nuts and seeds (especially pumpkin seeds), also may have a beneficial effect on alleviating the stubborn ailment. Sufferers should also make sure they are getting enough zinc and should drink as little alcohol and coffee as possible.

The original source of the news about Dr. Hernuss's remarkable experience with pollen is *Strahlentherapie* 150, number 5 (1975). This is a German magazine devoted to radiotherapy. The results, however, were abstracted in the April 1976 issue of *Prevention*. An article on pollen in the January 1977 *Let's Live* mentions a U.S. Department of Agriculture research project that showed that pollen inhibited the development of mammary tumors in laboratory animals.

The work by Deig and Ehresman in kelp was reported in *Time*, June 21, 1976. The role of both kelp and pectin in combating the effects of strontium 90 is discussed in an article in *Prevention*, December, 1974.

Sarah Harriman's well-documented *The Book of Ginseng* (Pyramid, 1976) is the source of much of my material on that provocative plant. Adams and Murray's *Health Foods* also contains some reliable data. I also drew on an article on ginseng published in the September 1973 issue of *Science et vie*. Dr. Cha's accidental discovery at Brown University was reported in a letter by Curt Norris in the *Smithsonian* magazine.

For more details on the periwinkle plant and cancer, see an article by Fred L. Shaw, Jr., in *Drug Topics*, July 27, 1964. As this book goes to press, much attention is being given to a plant called maytansine. Growing on vines near the Kenya Coast, maytansine has long been used by African witch doctors to treat cancer. It appears to have some genuine anticancer properties, and in 1977 the National Cancer Institute began testing it on terminal cancer patients.

For details on Dr. Berman's project see his *The Boston Police Diet and Weight Control Program* published in New York by Richard Fell. The American Cancer Society's rather startling discovery of lower heart attacks among egg eaters has been cited in numerous health publications. Adams and Murray discuss it along with other research on this subject in their above-cited book *Health Foods*. The monograph that Dr. Altschule wrote for *Executive Health* is entitled "The Much-Maligned Egg" and was published in 1974. This was two years before the publication of the Tecumseh, Michigan, study which, of course, virtually proved his point.

In my notes I find further references to other research and opinion along these lines. As far back as 1953 the *Journal of Mt. Sinai Hospital* in New York reported finding that although blood cholesterol levels rose immediately after consumption of a quantity of eggs, in a few hours the blood levels were back to where they had been before the eggs were eaten. Dr. Michael DeBakey once reported that an evaluation of 1,700 patients suffering hardening of the arteries showed no definitive relationship between their arterial problems and their cholesterol levels. And Dr. J. A. Carnie, a British biochemist, states in the May 26, 1976, *Lancet* that "there is almost no evidence that the amount of cholesterol in food influences the amount in the blood."

Chapter 7: Other Weapons, Other Ways

Rodale's book was published by Rodale Press in 1970. The various research studies on psychology and cancer were summarized by Mary G. Marcus in "Cancer and Character" in *Psychology Today*, June 1976, and by Dr. Elizabeth M. Whelan in "Stress and Cancer" in *Harper's Bazaar*, July 1976.

Later studies confirm the results of the earlier research reported in these two articles. For example, two psychologists report in the October, 1976, *Journal of Clinical Psychology* of a study of eighty-eight persons, of whom forty-four were suffering from various types of cancer and forty-four were afflicted with medical problems other than cancer. The two psychologists were not told beforehand which ones had the cancer. In interviewing and compiling the psychological case histories of the eighty-eight patients, the researchers found that those having cancer had, on the average, sustained twice as many emotionally upsetting events in their lives as the noncancer group.

Those wishing to obtain further information on the relation of psychology to cancer might wish to consult *You Can Fight For Your Life* by Lawrence LeShan (M. Evans & Co., 1977). In this book, psychologist LeShan describes in detail his own extensive work with cancer patients. It is regrettable, however, that so few psychiatrists, who are, of course, M.D.'s, have become interested in using their combined credentials to treat and, hopefully, to prevent cancer.

I should also like to pass on two other bits of data that might prove provocative for those wishing to probe further into this area. One study that I once came across showed that the cancer rate of schizophrenics was less than half that of the general population. And a study done in Greece revealed that the cancer mortality rate for incarcerated mental patients was only one-third that of the general population of that country. There would seem to be a fruitful field here for further investigation.

Dr. Simonton's work has been written up quite extensively. One informative article on this approach appeared in the January 1976 *Prevention*. The pharmaceutical firm Hoffman-La Roche is now making available to medical practitioners some educational tape recordings on the use of psychological healing methods. Meanwhile, psychologist LeShan has also trained over one hundred fifty people, including thirty-five doctors, with such methods.

One additional item on mind versus cancer may also be of interest. On August 22, 1976, the *Boston Globe* reported on a Massachusetts General Hospital study showing what kinds of cancer patients live longest. The study found that those patients who were angry and more demanding, as well as those who cooperated more fully with the medical staff, fared better in the hospital. Those who fared least well were those who were resigned to illness and death. (The study also showed that patients whose parents were often absent during their childhood and patients who had histories of unsatisfactory relationships with other people tended to die quicker. These findings tend to confirm those of the other studies cited above.)

For the material on meditation I have drawn on my own experience (I took a TM course) and also on a brief interview I had with Dr. Benson in the fall of 1975. Dr. Benson's valuable book *The Relaxation Response* is available in paperback (Avon, 1976). The report on the yoga experiments by the

Indian doctors was carried in the *New York Times,* November 30, 1975.

Much of the information on long-lived people who kept physically active comes from one of Dr. Roger Williams's earlier books, *Nutrition in a Nutshell* (Dolphin Books, 1962). Recently much more information has come to light on this subject. An exhaustive study by the California State Health Department and the University of California at Berkeley pretty much proved that people holding physically active jobs suffer fewer heart attacks than those practicing more sedentary occupations. (The study was reported in the "News of the Week in Review" of the *New York Times,* March 27, 1977).

A new and, for our purposes, much more important study comes from the Labor Science Research Institute in Japan. There, according to the February 1977 *Prevention,* mice given a carcinogen (benzidine) suffered substantially less cancer when an exercise wheel was put in their cage. Only 63 percent of the mice contracted cancer versus 93 percent of a control group that received the cancer-causing chemical but did not receive the exercise. As far as I know, this is the first experiment ever done linking cancer directly to exercise.

Exercise enthusiasts will take heart at this new evidence; however, they should still proceed with caution. President Eisenhower suffered his heart attack after playing 27 rounds of golf; the Reverend Gil Dodds, known as the "perambulating parson" for having broken the indoor mile track record, died of a stroke in February 1977 at the age of 58; and a one-time all-American football player from Michigan State has told me that half of his football team did not live to sixty-five. Physical activity does build health, but strenuous and competitive exercise can promote problems. Competitive exercise for some people probably creates more stress than it alleviates. (I have noticed that while tennis and golf players frequently seem to suffer heart attacks, those who folk dance appear to fare much better. Could it be due to the fact that successful folk dancing rests on cooperation rather than competition? This is an interesting area for further research.)

In *Nutrition in a Nutshell*, Dr. Roger A. Williams lists many of the benefits of breast-feeding over bottle-feeding. The July 4, 1976, issue of *Parade* quotes a professor of pediatric medicine, Dr. Derrick Jelliffe, as saying, "If our women knew what they were doing to their children by refusing to nurse, they would be ashamed." More recently there have been reports of increasing infant mortality rates in underdeveloped countries where bottle feeding has begun to supplant breast feeding.

The case against Laetrile is ably summed up in "Laetrile: The Making of a Myth," *FDA Consumer*, December 1976–January 1977. *Prevention* carried articles putting Laetrile in a more favorable light in its April 1972 and May 1974 issues. Also see Krebs's letter in the magazine's April 1972 issue. The United Nations study of the cancer-free Hunzas can be found in "Impact of Science on Society," published by the United Nations Educational, Social and Cultural Organization. The study was done by two Belgian scientists, Doctors Emile-Gaston Peeters and Yola Verhasselt. Dr. Rubin's preliminary findings were reported in *The News World*, May 11, 1977. On May 23, 1977, the National Cancer Institute announced that it was planning to seek approval to test Laetrile on humans.

The material regarding the questionable utility of regular check-ups as a means of cancer control comes from an article by Richard Spark, M.D., entitled "The Case against Regular Physicals" in the *New York Times Magazine*, July 25, 1976. The experience of Mrs. Nelson Rockefeller would seem to substantiate Dr. Spark's conclusion. The former vice president's wife was operated on for breast cancer in 1974. It appears that she first noticed a lump on her breast just two weeks after she had had a complete physical that had found her to be in good health.

Chapter 8: What Killed Adelle Davis?

An article on Winfield Franklin's formidable feat appeared in *Let's Live*, February 1974. The information on J. I. Rodale came from an article in *Prevention*, January 1975. Betty Lee Morales cast some revealing light on some little-known aspects of Adelle Davis's life and life-style in "Adelle's Last Days," *Let's Live*, July 1976.

Let's Get Well was published by Harcourt Brace Jovanovich in 1965, and a paperback edition was put out by the New American Library in 1972. The earlier Davis work cited is *Let's Eat Right to Keep Fit*, which was issued by the same publishers, the first edition appearing in 1954, the revised edition in 1970.

A report on Dr. Berg's paper can be found in the *New York Times*, December 3, 1975. On October 18 of the previous year, the *Times*, in connection with reporting the mastectomies of Mrs. Ford and Mrs. Rockefeller, carried a similar story. This one, written after interviewing various specialists in the field, pointed to meat and meat fat as prime causes of cancer of the breast. It was noted that Japan, where the diet is low in meat fat, has a remarkably low incidence of breast cancer. But when Japanese women migrate to the United States and start to consume an American diet, their incidence of breast cancer rises.

The Los Angeles study on polyunsaturates and cancer was summarized in *Prevention*, October 1972. For Dr. Harman's studies, see *Nutrition Today*, January 1972 and *Critical Reviews in Food Technology*, September 1972. Also the *New*

England Journal of Medicine of January 4, 1973, carried a report by three physicians indicating that people on a polyunsaturated diet were more than twice as likely to develop gallstones as those on a regular American diet.

Dr. Altschule's observations come from his report "How Much Do You 'Know' That Isn't So About Saturated vs. Polyunsaturated Fats?" *Executive Health* 10, number 10 (1974). Lest it be thought that Dr. Altschule, despite his impeccable credentials, stands alone in his judgments, I should like to call attention to the editorial board of *Executive Health*, which presumably approves all its publications. This board includes some of the most distinguished names in the medicinal-nutritional field.

The study on rats, fats, and bowel cancer was disclosed at the annual meeting of the American Society for Microbiology in New Orleans. It was reported in the *Boston Globe*, May 12, 1977, and quite probably in other newspapers of the same date.

For Dr. Leaf's assessments of protein consumption in the three long-life areas of the world, see his article in the January 1973 *National Geographic*. Another physician, who is also a biochemist, Michael M. Berman, has studied the people in the Russian region more intensively. Dr. Berman, who directed a health clinic in the USSR for fourteen years, says the Russian group eats meat only about once a week, and then it is usually lamb. Thus, it would seem that their protein intake might well fall below Dr. Leaf's estimates. (For a report on Berman's findings see an article by Jane Kinderlehrer in the February 1977 *Prevention*.) The final results of the Seventh Day Adventist study were reported in the *New York Times*, December 13, 1976. The *National Inquirer* of February 24, 1977, reported research done by a New York pediatrician that supports this earlier study. Dr. Allan S. Cunningham of Mary Imogene Bassett Hospital in Cooperstown, New York, had found cancer of the lymph linked to animal protein consumption in a fifteen-country survey. The newspaper also quoted Dr. Nathan Pritikin, head of the Longevity Research Institute in Santa Barbara, California, as confirming this conclusion. Pritikin claims that his institute has found that a high intake of animal protein correlates with a higher death rate not only from lymphoma but from other types of cancer as well.

The Australian study of vegetarian women was cited in an article by Peter Barry Chowka in the March 1977 *East West Journal*. The same issue of this magazine has articles by Gloria Swanson, in which she describes her experiences with Dr. Bieler, and by William Dufty, her husband, in which he reports the account of Dr. Moerman regarding the German occupation of Holland.

The first theory concerning how protein could cause problems is cited by Dr. Benjamin Frank in his previously examined book on nucleic acid. The amyloid theory is cited by Dr. Paalo Airola in his *Let's Live* column of June 1975. The subsequent quote from Dr. Airola is from the same column. The third theory is referred to by Geoffrey T. Whitehouse, D.S.C., F.R.S.H., in his book *Why Health Foods?* (Here's Health, 1968).

Fredericks's comment on protein's causing mineral loss is based on research reported in *Medical Tribune*, May 9, 1973. *Medical World News* of November 16, 1973, carried a story about fears of vitamin A deficiency from high-protein food sent to Upper Volta. Dr. G. Edwin Bunce has told of such deficiencies occurring in Brazil when relief organizations sent in high protein food following a famine in *Natural History*, February 1969. Dr. Nelson's observations can be found in *Medical World News*, November 8, 1974.

Dr. Denham Harman, in an article written by him in the February 1977 *Prevention* reports finding that vegetable protein substituted for animal protein in the diets of laboratory mice increased their life span. In this article he also reported that the life span of mice was also increased as the amount and/or degree of *unsaturation* of the fat in their diets was reduced. It is interesting to observe that this well-respected researcher—he is, after all, both a professor of medicine and a professor of biochemistry at the University of Nebraska College of Medicine—wrote the article for *Prevention* himself. This may be an indication of the growing respectability of magazines once sneered at as simply journals for health nuts.

There are a few other items worthy of note regarding protein, especially animal protein, and human health. *Nutrition* (1974) reported the case of a British teacher whose malignant melanoma of the left eye substantially regressed as a result of a diet low in two of the protein-building amino acids (tryosine and phenylalanine). Though rare, melanoma is a quite vicious and virulent form of cancer. It has a cure rate of less than 25 percent when standard treatments are followed.

High meat consumption has also been associated with other ailments. One Harvard research team has found a direct and close relationship between meat and high blood pressure, as reported in the *American Journal of Epidemiology*, November 1974. Many doctors warn of possible kidney problems from high protein consumption. And one physician who went on a high protein diet to reduce told me that while she did lose weight, she also became ill. Other people she knew who went on a similar diet for the same reason experienced similar problems. She pointed out that protein produces ammonia in the system.

Dr. Howell's article on beef and bowel cancer appeared in the *Journal of Chronic Diseases* 28 (1975). Dr. Shamberger's findings are well summarized in the August 1975 *Prevention*.

Assays of salt content in raw and canned peas and other foods can be found in *Composition of Foods*, Handbook Number 8, U.S. Department of Agriculture. All told, the average American consumes about 2.5 pounds of salt a year.

One research physician, Dr. Lewis K. Dahl, the late chief of staff at the Brookhaven National Laboratories, claims this is *forty times* as much as an adult needs to be healthy. Dr. Yudkins's book was published in this country by P.H. Wyden in 1972. Dr. Walford's study was summarized in *Nature's Way*, October 1973. There have been many other studies linking low dietary intake with longevity in laboratory animals. For example, the *Boston Herald American* of June 7, 1976, reported an experiment that showed that both rhesus monkeys and mice given controlled diets lived 33 percent longer than similar animals who ate what they wanted. For an interesting piece on how this principle may apply to man see *Executive Health* 4, number 5. For the caloric consumption in the three long-life regions, see Dr. Leaf's previously cited article in the *National Geographic*.

Dr. Cheraskin's observations on sugar and stress, along with Dr. Pfeiffer's concurrence, can be found in the July 1976 issue of *Let's Live*. The studies linking sugar and reduced resistance can be found in the *Journal of the California State Dental Association* 32, number 9 (1964) and the *American Journal of Clinical Nutrition* 26, number 2 (1973). For a more recent study, see Ringsdorf et al., *Dental Practice*, December 1976. Finally, a California physician, Edward R. Pinckney, M.D., claims that "sugar alone can stimulate the production of fat in the body," and we have already seen how fat can contribute to cancer. (Dr. Pinckney's statement is contained in his book *The Cholesterol Controversy*, published by Sherbourne Press in 1973. In this book Dr. Pinckney scores the drive to promote polyunsaturates as an aid to the heart. He covers many of the points we have already examined but adds one or two new ones. For instance he claims that scientists at the U.S. Agricultural Research Service have discovered that corn oil, the highly touted staple of margarine, actually produces *more* cholesterol than butter.)

The Wisconsin research on saccharin and cancer was

reported in *Science*, June 5, 1970. The Canadian studies, and the FDA's saccharin ban, which was based upon them, were written up in newspapers across the country on March 10, 1977. Dr. Marble's rebuttal was contained in an article he wrote for the *Boston Sunday Globe*, April 10, 1977. Carlton Fredericks cites as the source for his suggestion some research reported in the *Journal of Agricultural and Food Chemistry* (21:916).

For the role of coffee in bladder cancer see *Lancet*, June 26, 1975, and *Preventive Medicine*, number 2, 1973. Also see a column by Jean Mayer in the May 30, 1976, *Boston Globe*, which reports two studies done at Harvard that seem to confirm such a correlation. However, Mayer also claims that Canadian researchers found no such relationship.

For the UCLA research on beer consumption and cancer see the *Journal of the National Cancer Institute*, September 1977. The September 21, 1974, issue of *Lancet* reports research done at a Glasgow hospital showing that vitamin C helped remove alcohol from the blood. The more vitamin C the imbiber consumed, the faster the alcohol disappeared. Dr. Williams's research was also originally reported in *Lancet*.

My list of celebrities who puffed on cigars, pipes, or both well into their eighties and even nineties was drawn up quickly from memory and is certainly not meant to be exhaustive. It originally included Sigmund Freud, the cigar-smoking founder of modern psychotherapy. But Freud, so I later learned, did die of mouth cancer. It is interesting to note, however, that Freud's cancer did not flare up until he finally fled Vienna, a city that he loved, and went to live in England. It seems likely that this stressful move, brought on by the Nazi occupation of his country, had a good deal to do with his death from cancer soon after. He lived to eighty-three.

One further admonition for those who insist on smoking

cigarettes. When you are not actually puffing on it, do not hold the cigarette between your lips in Humphrey Bogart fashion. Doing that only increases the amount of smoke going into your lungs. It may be that the greater tendency of men smokers to do this is partly responsible for their greater lung cancer rate.

Regarding wine, a report in *Science News* of February 26, 1977, indicates that this drink may actually be something of a boon to health. Some new research shows that grapes and grape products contain compounds that have an antiviral activity. Several viruses were found to be destroyed when added to various extracts and infusions made from grapes. Wines were among the grape products tested. Red wines seem to be more potent in this respect than white wines, and this may be due to the fact that red wines are fermented with the skins. For more on this see Carlton Fredericks's column in *Prevention*, May 1977. For another report on the possibly positive effects of wine see *Executive Health* 8, number 3.

Dr. Fisher's remarks appeared in a symposium on facial care conducted by *Vogue* in 1976. Dr. Aimes's report on hair dyes and cancer can be found in *New Scientist*, March 27, 1975. For reports on the work of Dr. Weisberger and Dr. Shafer see *Prevention*, August 1975.

Dr. Saffiotti's findings were mentioned by Representative James J. Delaney of New York in remarks published in the *Federal Register* of February 9, 1972. For Dr. Berg's report on cancer-causing substances in water see *Internal Medicine News*, February 15, 1972. Meanwhile a new danger from water has arisen. On May 11, 1977, the *Washington Post* reported that the amount of chlorine added to water also seems to correlate with cancer, especially bladder cancer. The newspaper claimed that the U.S. Environmental Protection Agency had found this to be true. A spokesman at the agency subsequently confirmed this but added that the study was not yet completed and no definitive conclusions could be drawn.

Of the cities surveyed, Miami was found to have the highest chlorine content in its water.

The question of whether fluorine can cause or contribute to cancer remains an ongoing controversy. American medical and dental authorities generally maintain that the small amounts added to drinking water to foster dental health do not endanger any other part of the body. However, Dr. Dean Burk claims that fluoridation of water supplies in this country has killed half a million people over the past twenty-five years. "Fluoride," says Dr. Burk, "affects the intestinal tract, the kidneys, causes breast cancer, and as years go on, it affects every organ." (Dr. Burk's remarks were reported in *East West*, March 1977.) It will be recalled that he had earlier resigned as head of the cytochemistry section of the National Cancer Institute in a dispute over Laetrile.

The quote from Dr. Collins comes from Whiteside, *Why Health Foods?* For further success stories see the publications listed under the bibliographical notes and comments for chapter 2. Most of these people who cured themselves through dietary means ate food that could be called organic. However, I would like to echo Dr. Vachon's warning that most people would do well not to neglect other forms of therapy.

For data on DES and cancer see articles by Dr. Arthur L. Herbst in the *New England Journal of Medicine*, April 22, 1971, and in the *Journal of the American Medical Association*, May 1, 1972. For data on estrogen and cancer see Carlton Fredericks's column in *Prevention*, June 1974. He lists seven different research reports establishing such a link. For later research see the *New England Journal of Medicine*, December 4, 1975. This issue carries two articles on this subject plus an editorial that offers the hypothesis "that one might take estrogens for valid medical indications with a potential risk of cancer comparable to the self-abuse of over-eating or smoking."

The information from the International Commission on Radiological Protection comes from *Prevention*, November 1972, and the quote by Dr. Gofman is taken from the December 1973 issue of the same magazine. In July 30, 1973, the *Journal of the American Medical Association* published research implicating radiation in the development of cancer of the thyroid.

Chapter 9: Living the Anticancer Life

Pauling's statement regarding vitamin A is quoted in the April 1973 *Prevention*. In regard to Whipple's experiences, a report in the *Medical World News* of September 8, 1972, may be of interest. In this story Dr. Whipple tells of one of his early patients who, when cured of anemia, continued eating over a half pound of liver every single day. At the time the report appeared she was eighty years old and enjoying excellent health. Since she was ingesting over 100,000 units of vitamin A daily from her liver intake alone, this would seem to minimize any dangers that high vitamin A consumption can create *as long as the vitamin is in its natural form*.

The scarce report on vitamin C destroying vitamin B_{12} appeared in the October 14, 1974, *Journal of the American Medical Association*, and the contradicting report from the Saint Louis Hospital was published in the April 21, 1975, issue of the same magazine. It should also be pointed out that liver, which contains large amounts of vitamin B_{12}, also contains vitamin C. Thus, the two seem to coexist quite amicably.

For the source of Dr. Butterworth's assurances see the notes on chapter 3. I also think it worth noting again that Doctors Pauling, Szent-Gyorgyi, and Klenner are all over seventy—Szent-Gyorgyi is in his mid-eighties—and none of them show anything but good effects from their high vitamin C intake.

The vitamin E test done by the National Institute of Health was reported in the *American Journal of Clinical Nutrition* for December 1975. Dr. Ayers's statement was made in the form of a letter to the June 2, 1973, *Journal of the American Medical Association*. Dr. Jennings's book was published by Charles C. Thomas. A good article summarizing a lot of scientific research and opinion on the greater effectiveness of natural vitamins appeared in the June, 1974, *Prevention*. The quote from Dr. Forman comes from Whiteside, *Why Health Foods?* while Dr. Kadans' statement comes from his book *Encyclopedia of Fruits, Vegetables, Nuts and Seeds for Healthful Living* (Parker Publishing Co., 1973).

Regarding the interrelationships of food supplements, Dr. John Prutting, a member of the medical board of Doctor's Hospital in New York, points out that hospitalized patients found to have vitamin deficiencies continued to remain deficient after those vitamins were given them by injection. It was only after magnesium was added to the injections that the deficiencies cleared up. This was reported in *Family Circle*, March 3, 1971.

There have been a variety of studies showing that high consumption of high-fiber bread is a sound way to lose weight. For example, Dr. Hans Kaunitz of the Columbia University College of Physicians and Surgeons found that overweight patients not only shed excess poundage but kept it off as long as their intake of high-fiber bread remained high. The *Lancet* of December 22, 1973, carried an article by Dr. K. W. Heaton of the British Royal Infirmary explaining how this occurs. (Dr. Heaton also claims that sugar, even if consumed in small amounts, will add unneeded and unwanted pounds.) However, do not look for sensational and speedy weight losses with this method. They will take place only gradually over a period of time.

For an interesting article on the benefits of potatoes see "World's Most Versatile Vegetable" by Harmon Tupper in the March 1968 issue of *American Agriculturalist and the Rural New Yorker.* Tupper compares potatoes to bananas in that they "have a high satiety value and impart a full-stomach feeling that checks over-eating. Sodium content is so slight that the American Heart Association recommends them for low-salt diets."

The August 1974 issue of *Prevention* contained an informative article on chili as a health food. Chili peppers are apparently rich storehouses of vitamins A and C. What's more, research conducted at the New Mexico State University shows that red chili acts as an antioxidant and helps preserve meats and fats from becoming rancid. And research conducted at the Max Planck Institute has shown, says *Prevention*, that "certain aromatic substances such as chili can promote the circulation of blood through the peripheral vessels of the skin and also lower the density of the coagulation compound."

Chocolate bars, even with almonds, are certainly best avoided. Chocolate not only requires heavy amounts of sugar to overcome its naturally bitter taste but also contains substantial amounts of fat. Chocolate contains two stimulants, caffeine and theobromine, as well as an acid that may interfere with the body's absorption of calcium. Carob, a foodstuff that greatly resembles chocolate, makes a much more acceptable base for candies and other sweets. It contains no stimulants or harmful acids and has little fat. It is naturally sweet, which means that it requires less sugar supplementation, and it has some fiber and small amounts of minerals. Carob bars can be purchased in health food stores.

A still better form of candy is a Jewish treat known as halvah. Halvah is made from sesame seeds, which are, it will be remembered, top-notch suppliers of selenium. These seeds also contain lecithin, a compound that helps protect the heart. However, halvah still contains lots of sugar; so do not regard it as a health food. As for other sweets, pumpkin and squash pies are less injurious than most others since they not only contain some nutritious ingredients but also have only one layer of crust. And oatmeal, molasses, and peanut butter cookies are less harmful than most other cookies.

Returning to some of the more basic issues involved in diet and cancer, the interested reader may wish to look at an article entitled "New Clues to Cancer," which appeared in the January 1977 issue of *Atlas.* This magazine reprints what it regards as significant articles from the world press. This particular article was first published in the highly respected *Sunday Times* of London and was written by that newspaper's medical correspondent, Oliver Gillie.

Gillie starts out by indicting the rich diet that we affluent Westerners eat as a prime, if not the prime, source of our surging cancer rate. In drawing up his bill of particulars of our dietary regimen, he covers much of the material we have already examined. But he adds some interesting and important information. For example, not only do Japanese women living in the United States suffer from a four times greater rate of breast cancer than do their sisters in the home country, but the same differences also hold true for cancers of the ovary and bowel and, in men, of the prostate and testis. Not only does Argentina suffer from nearly as much bowel cancer as the United States and Great Britain, but it has almost as much breast cancer as well. Apparently beef can cause more than one type of cancer.

Israel, he says, "provides a striking demonstration of the dietary connection." Breast cancer is about three times as likely to strike an European Jew as an African or Asian Jew. This, says Gillie, "is almost certainly because European Jews bring with them affluent Western eating habits while Asian diets are more frugal." He also points out that girls who menstruate at an earlier age tend to have a higher cancer rate, and that a "rich diet" tends to bring on early menstruation. Women who have unusual menstrual problems, who are older when they have their first child, and who start their menopause later all show more vulnerability to breast cancer. Gillie mentions one rather striking piece of research that had not previously come to my attention. This study shows that the liver houses certain enzymes that inactivate cancer-causing substances. However, rats fed a highly purified diet were unable to make these enzymes *even though they received sufficient quantities of all known vitamins, minerals, and other nutrients*. It seems that they needed vegetables, especially fresh vegetables, to produce these enzymes. Simply adding alfalfa to their diet enabled them to do so.

The researcher, Dr. Leo Wattenberg of the University of Minnesota, also found a variety of other foods that stimulate the production of these crucial enzymes. They include cabbage, brussel sprouts, turnips, broccoli, cauliflower, spinach, dill, and celery. Citrus fruits, beans, and seeds also seemed helpful in protecting the body from cancer.

Says Gillie in summing up the results of all this research, "These new dietary theories could . . . have the biggest impact on health since the germ theory led to vaccines and health measures that have stamped out the most common fatal infections." Coming from the sober, staid *Times* of London, that is quite a statement.

One reason that nutrition becomes even more important to those already suffering from cancer is that most conventional cancer therapies, such as surgery, radiation and chemotherapy, reduce the patient's resistance. Writing in the February 1974 issue of *Let's Live*, Alan Nittler, M.D., points out that "one of the major hazards resulting from the administration of chemotherapeutic agents for cancer is their effect on the white blood cells. They can be knocked out so that they are not being produced in enough numbers to protect the body." Dean Burk, the controversial biochemist who once headed an important division of the National Cancer Institute, goes still further. He says not only that such drugs tend to destroy the patient's immunization system but that they are in themselves toxic at applied dosages and even carcinogenic! He made this assertion in a letter to the National Cancer Institute director, Dr. Frank Rauscher, which was quoted in *East West*, April 1977.

That improved nutrition can help those undergoing such unpleasant therapies is becoming more and more evident to the medical profession. Doctors Edward M. Copeland and Stanley L. Dudrick, both of Houston, have found that giving a cancer patient a full range of nutrients makes him stronger, more comfortable, and more able to recover. (This was reported in the January 1976 *Prevention*. The same article also reported on a letter signed by six British physicians that had recently appeared in a British medical magazine. The six British doctors claimed that when they gave their cancer patients a relatively simple and conservative treatment, they not only lived more comfortably but also lived longer than did patients who received "aggressive" therapy. Those wishing to find a physician who would be more responsive to such approaches might do well to consult the membership directory of the International Academy of Preventive Medicine. The directory is obtainable by sending $3.50 to the Academy at 10409 Town and Country Way, Suite 200, Houston, Texas 77024.)

Returning to the task of annotation, the quote from Dr. Williams is from *Nutrition Against Disease*; the material on Harvey, Semmelweis, and Pillemer is from Glasser, *The Body Is the Hero*. Dr. Gio Gori's statement first appeared in *The Real Paper* of March 31, 1976 (this is a weekly published in Cambridge, Massachusetts). Dr. Daro was written up in the June 1976 *Prevention*. Dr. Sabin's admonition was cited in Adams and Murray's *Body, Mind and the B Vitamins* (Larchmont, 1972). The figures on longevity today as compared to 1789 can be found in an article by Dr. Johan Bjorksten in the *Relevant Scientist* 1 (1971).

To end on an enheartening note, Dr. Theodore Cooper has admitted taking "fairly large doses" of vitamins C and B complex. He feels they increase his resistance to infections and produce other "interesting benefits" as well. And who is Dr. Theodore Cooper? He is the new assistant secretary for Health in the Department of Health, Education and Welfare. Thus, the nation's "top doctor" has at least started to move in what is for modern medicine a new direction. Let's hope many more of his colleagues will join him and soon!

Index

Index

Index